Surgery of Trismus in Oral Submucous Fibrosis

Madan Kapre • Sudhanshu Kothe
Editors

Surgery of Trismus in Oral Submucous Fibrosis

An Atlas

BYWORD BOOKS™

Springer

Editors
Madan Kapre
Neeti Clinics
Neeti Gaurav Complex
Nagpur, Maharashtra
India

Sudhanshu Kothe
Department of Plastic and Reconstructive Surgery
Jai Clinics and Neeti Clinics
Nagpur, Maharashtra
India

ISBN 978-981-10-4890-6 ISBN 978-981-10-4892-0 (eBook)
https://doi.org/10.1007/978-981-10-4892-0

Library of Congress Control Number: 2017953443

Printed on acid-free paper

Springer Nature Singapore is part of Springer Science+Business Media (www.springer.com)
Byword Books Private Limited, Delhi, India (www.bywordbooks.in)

Preface

Trismus due to oral submucous fibrosis is a specific condition involving the mouth. This is common in geographical areas where chewing of betel nut and tobacco is prevalent. We encounter this condition frequently in our practice in Central India. As the number of treated patients started to grow in the late 1990s and the early 2000s, we realized that our approach towards the management of this disorder was in the right direction. We successfully applied some new methods such as platysma flap and mandibular mucoperiosteal flaps to treat this trismus.

As experience grew, we established these protocols in our management and consolidated the surgical treatment of trismus. Our failures have been our greatest teachers and the source of our inspiration. This atlas puts forth our methods and techniques in the management of trismus due to oral submucous fibrosis. It sums up our work of over more than two decades, which started with steroid injections and small release procedures, and went on to become comprehensive releases with regional myocutaneous flap reconstructions.

This atlas describes our surgical techniques and is meant to help those surgeons who encounter these disorders. Very often one finds oneself in a rather helpless situation, as there is a scarcity of literature and didactic advice. This atlas will help them in creating their own protocols of management. The authors have objectively analyzed their own successes and failures with different techniques and given a clear message at the end of this atlas. The initial six chapters give details of how we deal with this disorder; in the following section each page has clinical photographs, with brief description below. The reader may choose to read the atlas as a textbook or as a reference work.

We are grateful to all our patients who gave us an opportunity to help them overcome their problems and to those clinicians who have worked in this field before us.

Nagpur, Maharashtra, India — Madan Kapre
Nagpur, Maharashtra, India — Sudhanshu Kothe

Contents

About the Editors

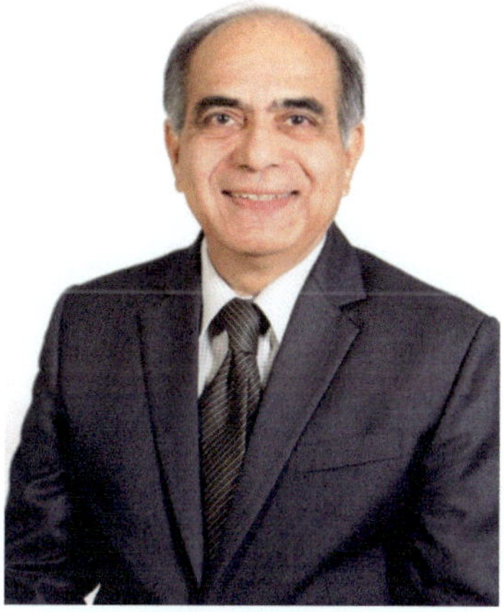

Madan Kapre F.R.C.S., D.L.O. is a consultant ENT and head and neck surgeon and former president of the Foundation for Head & Neck Oncology (FHNO), India. He is currently the managing director of Neeti Clinics, Nagpur, in Central India. He was trained in the UK and specializes in the surgery for trismus in OSMF. He is also an advisor to the Asia-Pacific Thyroid Society, Okinawa, Japan (email: madankapre@gmail.com).

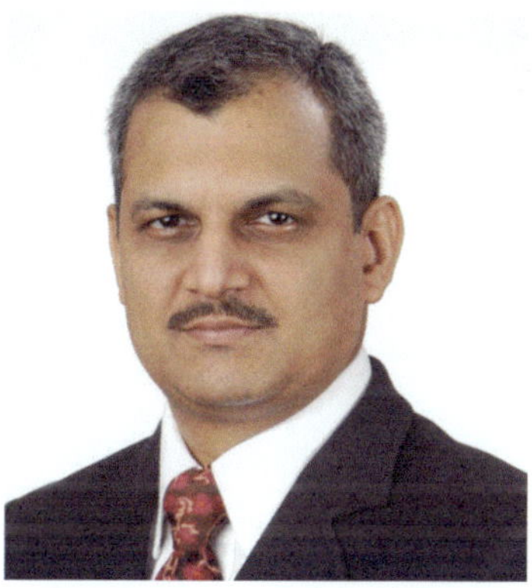

Sudhanshu Kothe M.S., M.Ch., D.N.B. is a consultant plastic and reconstructive surgeon at various clinics including Jai Clinics and Neeti Clinics, Nagpur, in Central India. He has a keen interest in reconstructive head and neck cancer microsurgery. His concept of using platysma myocutaneous flap has revolutionized the surgery for trismus in OSMF (email: sudhanshu.kothe@gmail.com).

Introduction: The Process of Trismus Due to Oral Submucous Fibrosis

1

Sudhanshu Kothe and Madan Kapre

Key Points

- Oral submucous fibrosis is a chronic condition.
- It affects not only submucosa of the oral cavity but also involves muscles, bones, and joints surrounding the affected area.
- Management of dental issues, infections, ulcers, and oral hygiene precedes surgical management of trismus.

Oral submucous fibrosis (OSMF) is a chronic condition of the mouth characterized by juxta-epithelial inflammatory reaction and progressive fibrosis of the submucosal tissues. The fibrosis progresses and affects tissues beyond the submucosa (muscles, bones, and joints), leading to rigidity and inability to open the mouth adequately (trismus). OSMF is considered a premalignant condition. The term oral submucous fibrosis was coined by Dr S.G. Joshi in 1953.

OSMF is associated with betel nut and quid chewing, a common practice in India.

Trismus is a sequel of advanced OSMF. The oral submucosa and mucosa is densely fibrosed, with significant contraction of tissues. The dimensions of all tissues eventually reduce. Muscles contract, lose length, and become fibrotic. The bones may become smaller, and joints may become contracted and lose mobility.

S. Kothe, M.S., M.Ch., D.N.B.
Department of Plastic and Reconstructive Surgery, Jai Clinics and Neeti Clinics, Nagpur, Maharashtra, India
e-mail: sudhanshu.kothe@gmail.com

M. Kapre, F.R.C.S., D.L.O. (✉)
Neeti Clinics, Neeti Gaurav Complex, Central Bazar Road, Ramdaspeth, Nagpur, Maharashtra, India
e-mail: madankapre@gmail.com

M. Kapre, S. Kothe (eds.), *Surgery of Trismus in Oral Submucous Fibrosis*,
https://doi.org/10.1007/978-981-10-4892-0_1

Oral opening reduces significantly in later stages, leading to poor oral hygiene. Gingival and dental infections are common, further leading to inflammation and fibrosis.

Cheeks lose stretchability and upper and lower sulci lose depth, eventually creating acute grooves, difficult to reach while cleaning. The tongue loses bulk, becomes fibrotic, and loses prehensility. It becomes difficult to reach the outer side of the teeth, and the vestibule, with the tongue. This leads to further deterioration of hygiene and eventually further fibrosis.

Contracture bands appear in the mucosa, tightening it. These bands suffer ulcerations and cracks, which get infected, and lead to inflammation and fibrosis. Introducing instruments for maintaining hygiene in the cheeks and oral cavity becomes difficult.

Muscles of mastication and the buccal and facial muscles lose bulk and undergo hypotrophy due to disuse. Fibrosis occurs in these muscles, and eventually they become tight bands.

Bones lose bulk and become weak. Temporomandibular joints suffer contraction and lose excursion, and the joint space eventually reduces in size. Movements of the jaws are reduced, and translation is lost significantly in the later stages of trismus.

Fibrosis may extend to the palatal mucoperiosteum and the soft palate. The soft palate becomes tight, contracted, and smaller in dimension. There may be ulcerations in the palatal mucosa. Uvula becomes contracted and small.

Bands of contracture may extend from soft palate through the retromolar mucosa to the mandibular area, leading to contraction and stiffness of the lower jaw.

Fibrosis may extend to the oropharynx to some extent.

Dental and gingival infections are common and lead to loss of teeth. The gingiva flattens away, and fibrotic ridges form on the alveolus.

In advanced stages, teeth abut against each other, and maxillary and mandibular incisors overlap.

Clinical Presentation

2

Madan Kapre and Sudhanshu Kothe

Key Points
- Trismus of OSMF origin has four grades, classified according to surgical planning.
- OSMF may involve all structures in the mouth and around.
- Anesthesia techniques are planned before surgery.
- It is important to identify symptoms that are NOT due to OSMF.

Under the restraint of the title of the book, general symptoms of OSMF, like burning in oral cavity, intolerance to temperature and spicy food, and general nutritional deficiency symptoms, are excluded. Authors shall restrict to the pathological changes in oral cavity responsible for trismus. The structures classically affected are the cheek, teeth, anterior tonsillar pillar and soft palate, muscles of mastication, and temporomandibular joint. Hence, the surgeon needs to address the dense hyalinized tissues in all these areas to achieve adequate release of trismus, i.e., to improve mouth opening.

The following pictures shall demonstrate all above and the factors that need to be considered before surgery.

M. Kapre, F.R.C.S., D.L.O. (✉)
Neeti Clinics, Neeti Gaurav Complex, Central Bazar Road, Ramdaspeth, Nagpur, Maharashtra, India
e-mail: madankapre@gmail.com

S. Kothe, M.S., M.Ch., D.N.B.
Department of Plastic and Reconstructive Surgery, Jai Clinics and Neeti Clinics, Nagpur, Maharashtra, India
e-mail: sudhanshu.kothe@gmail.com

M. Kapre, S. Kothe (eds.), *Surgery of Trismus in Oral Submucous Fibrosis*,
https://doi.org/10.1007/978-981-10-4892-0_2

Grades of Trismus

Grading is done strictly after 3 months of cessation of the injurious habits of chewing tobacco, areca nut, catechu mixed with lime, and similar offending habits.

Grades are measured in centimeters of inter-incisor distance (IID).

Grade 0: Symptoms of OSMF without trismus

Grade 1: Inter-incisor distance equal to or more than 3 cm

Grade 2: Inter-incisor distance between 2.9 and 2 cm

Grade 3: Inter-incisor distance between 1.9 and 1 cm

Grade 4: Inter-incisor distance less than 1 cm

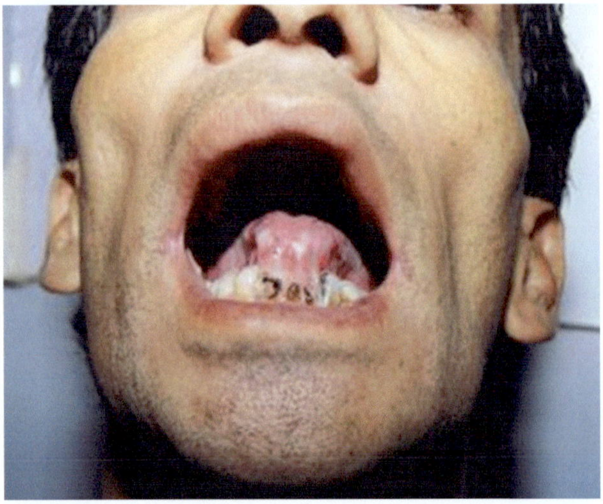

Fig. 2.1 OSMF involves the cheek, teeth, palate, floor of mouth, and occasionally the undersurface of the tongue, as in this picture

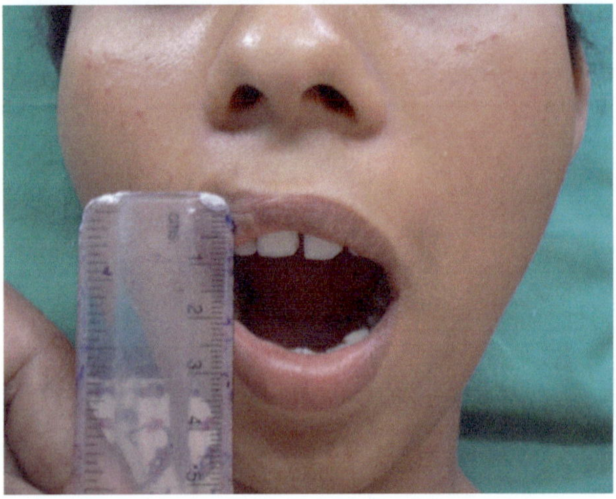

Fig. 2.2 Although this is not severe trismus, i.e., Grade 2 trismus (IID 2 cm), please note that this is a young female patient, and she will not like any facial scars. Hence, reconstruction will be restricted to procedures using intraoral tissues

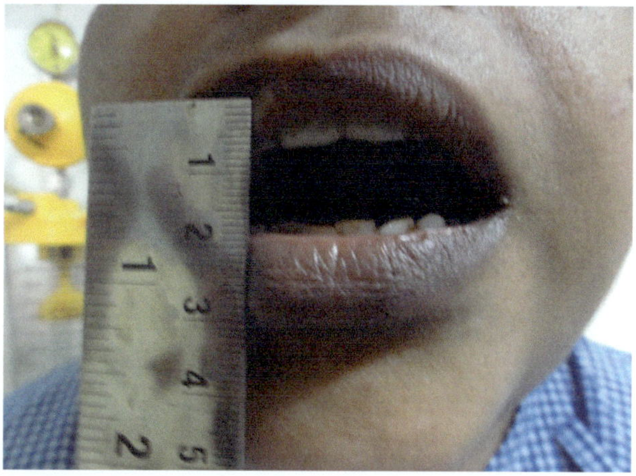

Fig. 2.3 This is Grade 3 trismus (IID 1.1 cm), in a young female. Hence, intraoral options of reconstruction desirable, i.e., fat, palatal flap, and mandibular mucoperiosteal flap (MMPF)

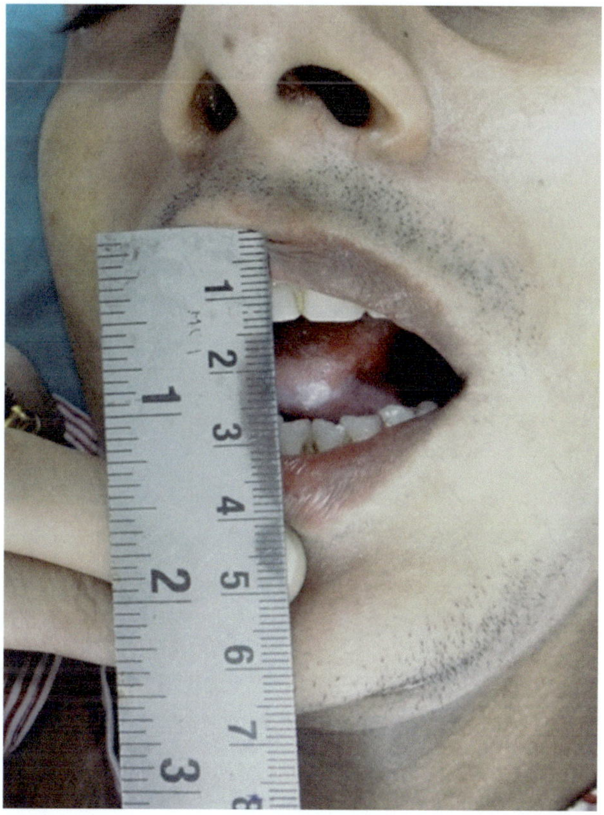

Fig. 2.4 Grade 3 trismus (IID 1.3 cm) in a young man and obviously extraoral choices for reconstruction are available, after counseling with patient, i.e., platysma myocutaneous flap

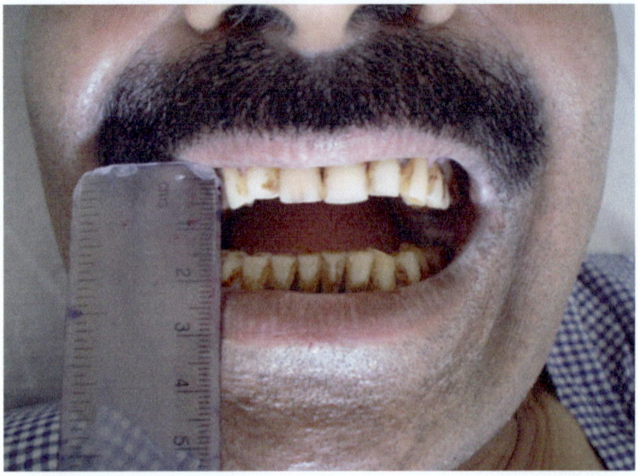

Fig. 2.5 Grade 4 trismus (IID 0.9 mm), in a short necked, stubby individual, hence there will be considerable difficulty in administering anesthesia. The anesthesiologist should be consulted and patient counseled together in a joint consultation

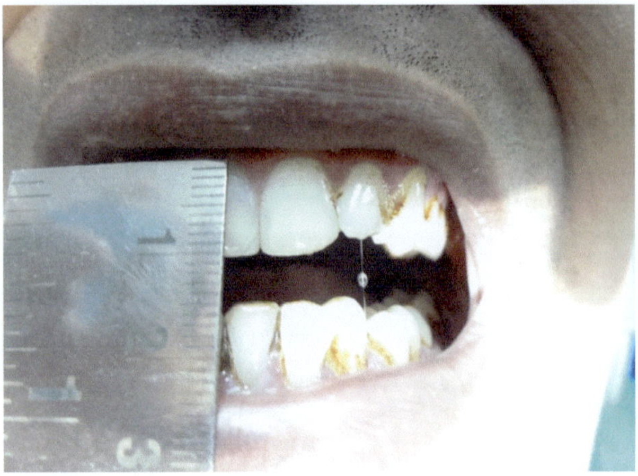

Fig. 2.6 Grade 4 trismus (IID 5 mm). Here, blind nasal intubation or endoscopically assisted intubation should be considered for administering anesthesia

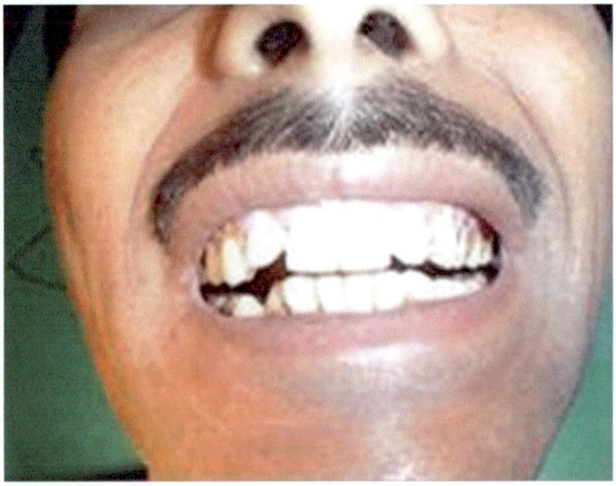

Fig. 2.7 Grade 4 trismus (IID 0 mm). In such severe cases, authors keep tracheostomy on the standby and execute it without hesitation. The tracheostomy can be removed intraoperatively at the end of the procedure

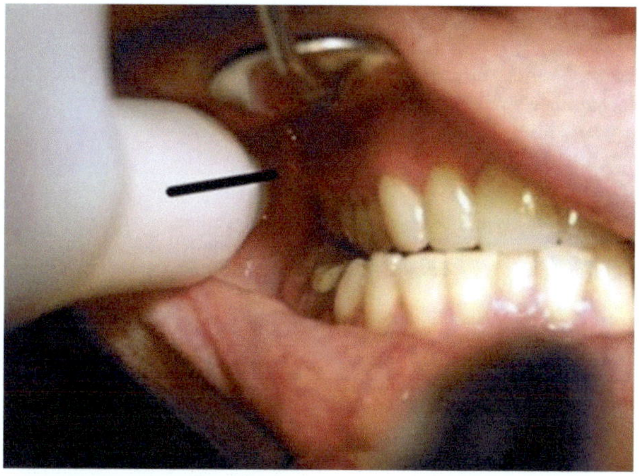

Fig. 2.8 Following are not the symptoms of trismus of OSMF: (1) halitosis, (2) pain, (3) bleeding, (4) falling teeth, (5) sudden increase in trismus, and (6) ulcerative growth in the retromolar area, as in this photograph

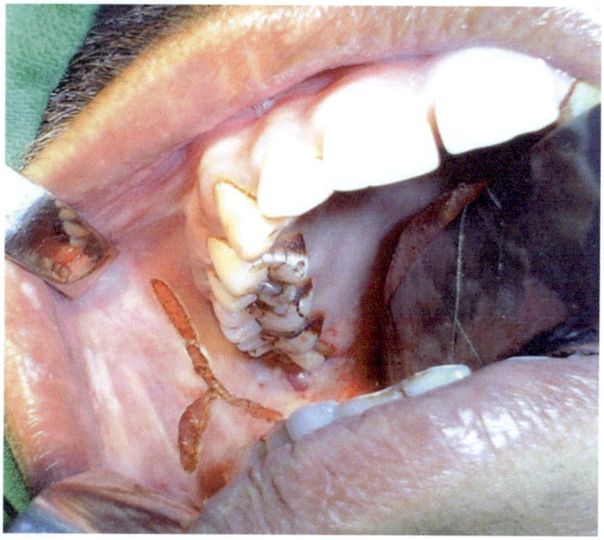

Fig. 2.9 This photograph classically demonstrates the three constricting bands causing trismus. (1) Just behind the oral commissure, (2) midway between commissure and retromolar area, and (3) retromolar area

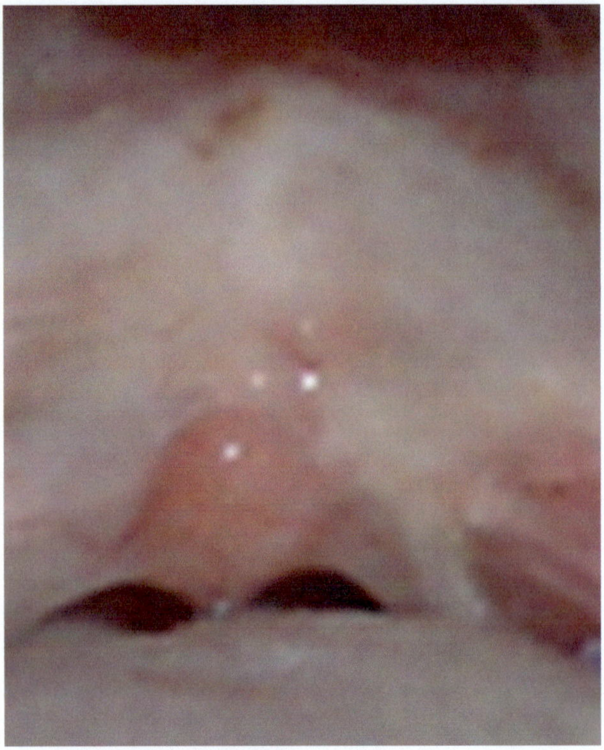

Fig. 2.10 Vesiculation, ulceration, that leads to burning mouth and intolerance shall continue unabated despite surgical treatment of trismus of OSMF. Upturned, contracted uvula due to OSMF is seen in this photograph

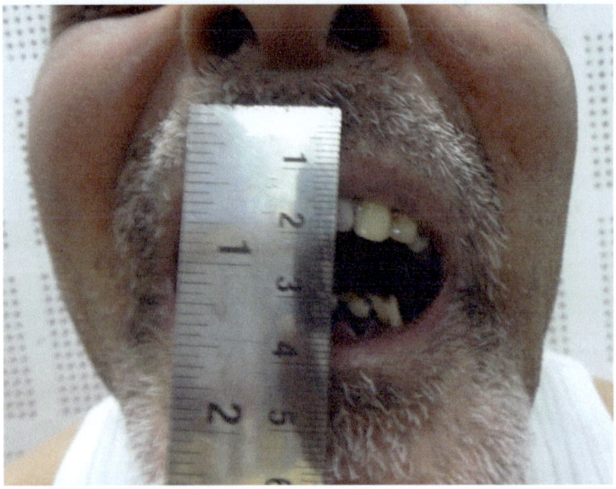

Fig. 2.11 Adequate attention has to be paid to dental hygiene, loose teeth and advancing age should warn the surgeon of lurking malignancy, which will demand thorough investigations and adequate counseling

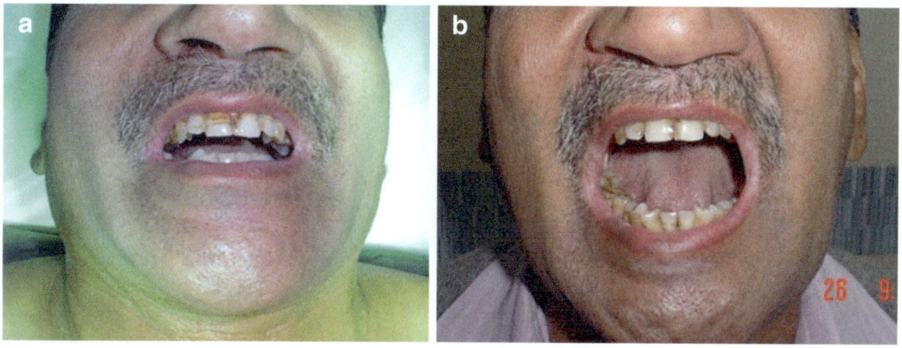

Fig. 2.12 (**a**, **b**) Strong motivation of the patient and good postoperative pain management and physiotherapy result in good outcomes

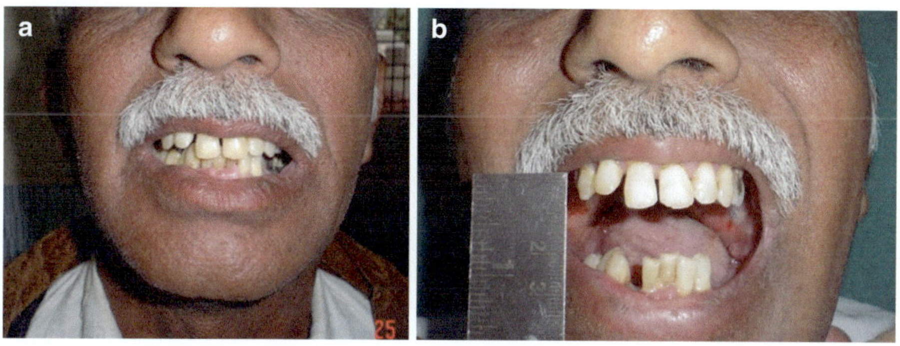

Fig. 2.13 (**a**, **b**) Lack of adequate motivation on the part of the patient, inadequate counseling and physiotherapy pain management, can lead to suboptimal results

Anesthesia for Surgery of Trismus Due to OSMF

3

Vidula Kapre

Key Points

The cornerstones in ensuring success for this elective surgical procedure are:

- Preoperative planning and preparation
- Prudence during induction
- Postoperative pain management

The approach is patient centric and well-coordinated team effort is very important.

Counseling of patients preoperatively is especially important in these cases.

Anesthesia plan is based on:

- Assessment of patient
- Skill of anesthesiologist
- Availability of resources

Awake intubation and bronchoscopy, or tracheostomy, are very useful techniques.

There should always be backup plans in case plan A fails. A strict dictum to be followed is never to administer muscle relaxant unless at least bag mask ventilation is assured.

V. Kapre
Neeti Clinics, Neeti Gaurav Complex, Central Bazar Road, Ramdaspeth,
Nagpur, Maharashtra, India
e-mail: vidulakapre@gmail.com

M. Kapre, S. Kothe (eds.), *Surgery of Trismus in Oral Submucous Fibrosis*,
https://doi.org/10.1007/978-981-10-4892-0_3

Assessment

Apart from routine assessment, these patients are assessed on the grade of trismus.

Anesthesiologist

Mechanism of securing the airway will be guided by the skill and expertise of anesthesiologist in performing various awake intubation techniques.

Resources

Fig. 3.1 Difficult Airway Cart

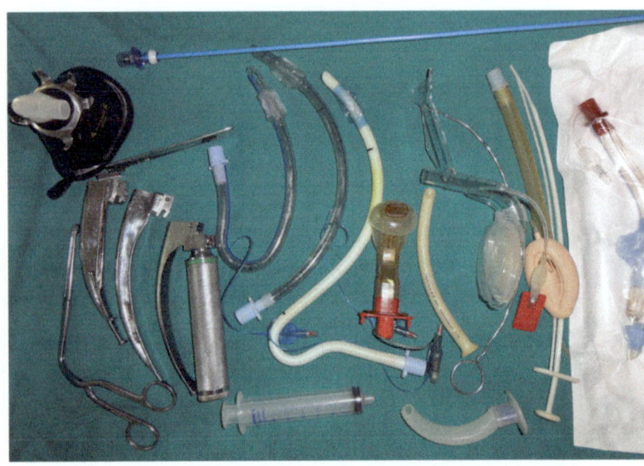

Difficult airway cart should be ready with each equipment in working condition. Point to be made here is that laryngeal mask airways or video laryngoscopes are of no use in these cases because of limited mouth opening. Flexible fiberoptic bronchoscope is the gold standard in case of awake intubation. Bonfils retromolar laryngoscope is useful but requires patient to be anesthetized.

Thus based on the above parameters, anesthesiologist should classify their approach toward securing the airway:

1. Routine induction and muscle relaxant—Grade I patients and Grade II patients where check laryngoscopy and bag mask ventilation before administering muscle relaxant are found to be satisfactory.
2. Anesthesia induction but no muscle relaxant—Grade II patients where check laryngoscopy and/or bag mask ventilation not satisfactory. Grades II, III, IV patients where Bonfil's laryngoscope is to be used.

3. Awake intubation is the method of choice for Grade IV patients. It can be:
   - Blind nasal intubation
   - Intubation with flexible fiberoptic bronchoscope
   - Retromolar intubation
4. Tracheostomy—Grade IV patients where either skill or resources for awake intubation not available or the patient is uncooperative.

Awake Intubation

Counseling

Premedication is given in the form of glycopyrrolate to reduce secretions, midazolam to allay anxiety, and fentanyl as analgesic but at half the dose so that respiratory efforts are not dampened. Air passage is anesthetized by:

- Nebulization with 4% lignocaine
- Bilateral superior laryngeal nerve blocks
- Transtracheal injection with 2% lignocaine

Nasal cavities are anesthetized and decongested with cotton patties soaked in 4% lignocaine with adrenaline.

In blind nasal technique intubation performed by constantly listening to breath sounds as the tube is gently advanced toward the trachea through the nose. At the point of maximum breath sounds, endotracheal tube is passed through the glottis during inspiration. A straight tube is always used for best conduction of breath sounds. Flexible fiberoptic bronchoscope is the gold standard. Endotracheal tube is loaded over the flexible scope. The scope is introduced through the nose and advanced toward the larynx under direct vision. As it passes beyond the vocal cords, tracheal rings are seen. The tube is then advanced into the trachea and the scope is withdrawn.

Innovations

Author shares her own innovations which are useful in Grades III and IV patients where fiberoptic bronchoscope is not affordable.

1. Not so blind intubation—Patient is prepared as for awake intubation. Endotracheal tube is advanced through the nose, but as against blind nasal intubation, the passage of the tube and the laryngeal inlet are visualized either with a flexible laryngoscope (1/4 cost of fiberoptic bronchoscope) introduced through other nostril or a 0° nasal endoscope introduced through retromolar space.

2. The other technique is useful in Grade III patients. Patient is preoxygenated and anesthetized, but no muscle relaxant is given. Endotracheal tube is introduced through the nose. Although mouth opening is limited, it can accept tip of laryngoscope blade. Here the laryngoscope is not used to visualize the larynx but to
   - Push the tongue in submandibular space.
   - Gentle rocking movement helps to advance the blade slightly, to allow tip of Magill forceps to be introduced.
   - Laryngoscope provides illumination to visualize the tube in the oropharynx, while Magill forceps is used to keep the tube in the midline as it is advanced toward larynx. Coughing and bucking by patient indicate that the endotracheal tube is in trachea. It is confirmed by auscultation and end-tidal CO_2.

Once airway is secure and surgery begins, the main concern is to provide good analgesia and depth of anesthesia to keep the heart rate and blood pressure low.

Above approach will ensure safe smooth anesthesia comfort to the patient and most important good surgical outcome.

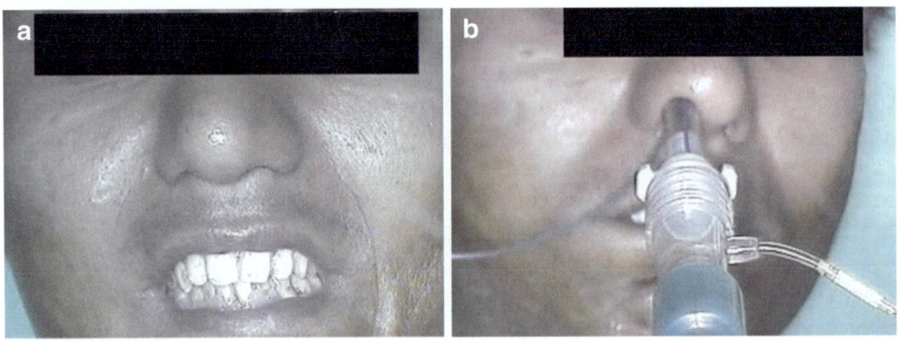

Fig. 3.2 (**a**, **b**) Awake blind nasal intubation

Awake Blind Nasal Intubation

Awake blind nasal intubation is a very useful skill for anesthesiologist, especially in noninstitutional setups where flexible fiberoptic bronchoscope is not affordable; proper counseling of patients to gain their confidence, calm and confident approach, and looking out for the patients' comfort ensure success without discomfort to the patients.

After preparing nasal passage and anesthetizing the airway, the endotracheal tube is lubricated with 2% jelly and introduced through the nose.

- The tube is gently advanced through nasopharynx and oropharynx.
- One ear of the anesthesiologist is at the upper end of the endotracheal tube, constantly listening to breath sounds.
- At the point of maximum breath sounds, the tube is directed anteriorly and downward to pass through the larynx.

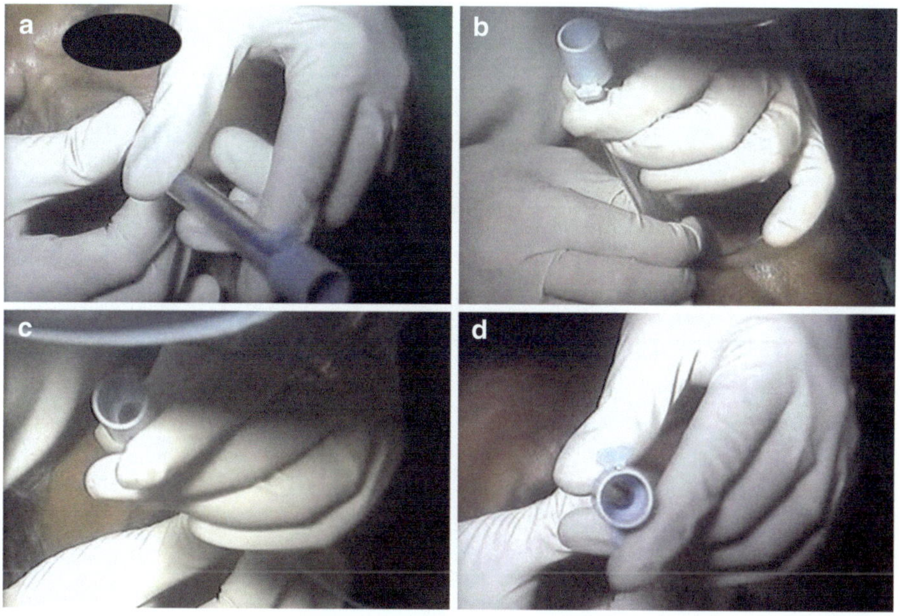

Fig. 3.3 (**a–d**) Nasal intubation: Introducing and guiding the tube

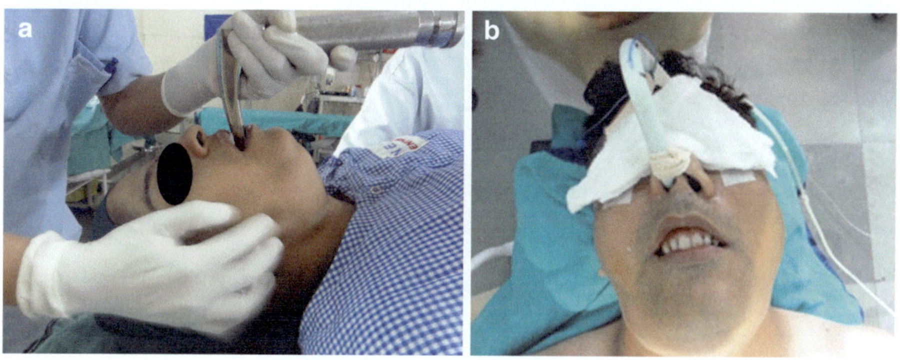

Fig. 3.4 (**a**, **b**) Nasal intubation: Introduction and fixation of tube

If mouth opening is < 20 mm, just sufficient to introduce tip of the laryngoscope blade and Magill forceps, nasal intubation is possible. The laryngoscope provides illumination within the oral cavity, and Magill forceps helps to advance the tube in midline (Fig. 3.1).

Difficult intubation kit should be well laid out with all equipment in working condition.

In Grade IV trismus patients, awake intubation can be aided by providing view of larynx either by flexible laryngoscope introduced through either nostril or 0° nasal endoscope introduced through retromolar space.

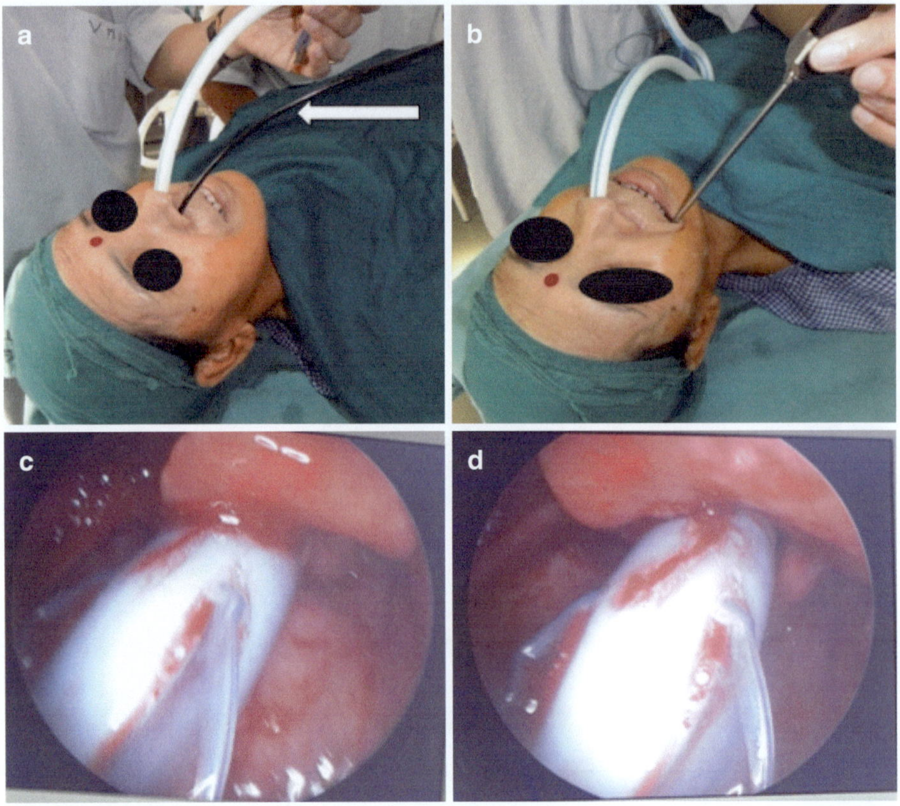

Fig. 3.5 (**a–d**) Use of endoscopy to aid awake intubation

Surgical Release Procedures for Trismus

4

Madan Kapre, Sudhanshu Kothe, and Neeti Kapre Gupta

Key Points

- Systematic release of contracted tissues is achieved by scalpel or laser.
- Each grade of trismus demands a different release procedure.
- Coronoidectomy is necessary in higher grades of trismus.

We strongly recommend that the surgical excision of scar tissue and division of bands, which are demonstrated in this chapter, should be carried out in a systematic orderly fashion on both sides in tandem. This will achieve gradual opening of the mouth to increase inter-incisor distance and minimize inadvertent damage to the teeth. This also avoids unintentional tears in the areas where tissues are precious and mucosa is scarce.

M. Kapre, F.R.C.S., D.L.O. (✉) • N.K. Gupta, M.S., D.N.B. (ENT)
Neeti Clinics, Neeti Gaurav Complex, Central Bazar Road, Ramdaspeth,
Nagpur, Maharashtra, India
e-mail: madankapre@gmail.com; neetikapregupta@gmail.com

S. Kothe, M.S., M.Ch., D.N.B.
Department of Plastic and Reconstructive Surgery, Jai Clinics and Neeti Clinics,
Nagpur, Maharashtra, India
e-mail: sudhanshu.kothe@gmail.com

M. Kapre, S. Kothe (eds.), *Surgery of Trismus in Oral Submucous Fibrosis*,
https://doi.org/10.1007/978-981-10-4892-0_4

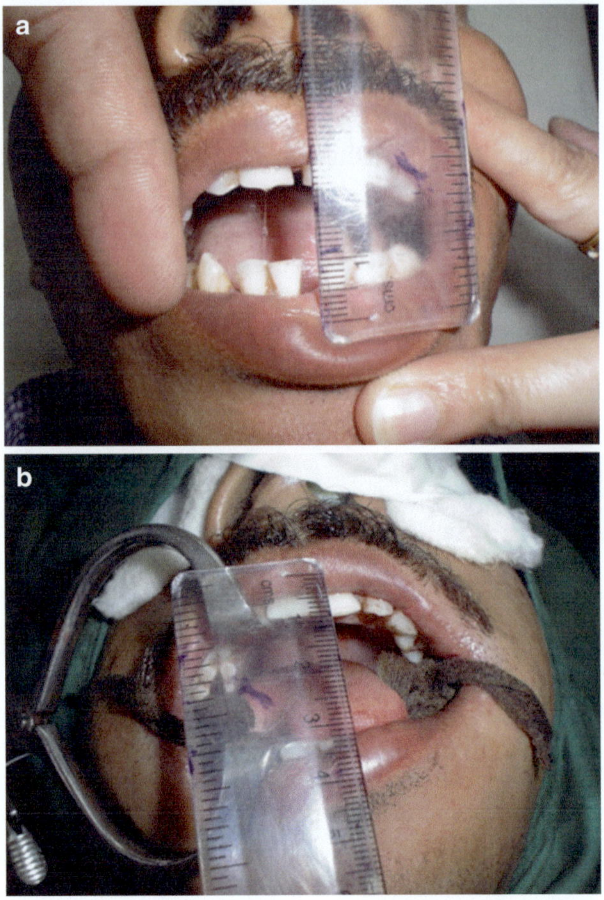

Fig. 4.1 (**a**, **b**) Measuring the interincisor distance before release

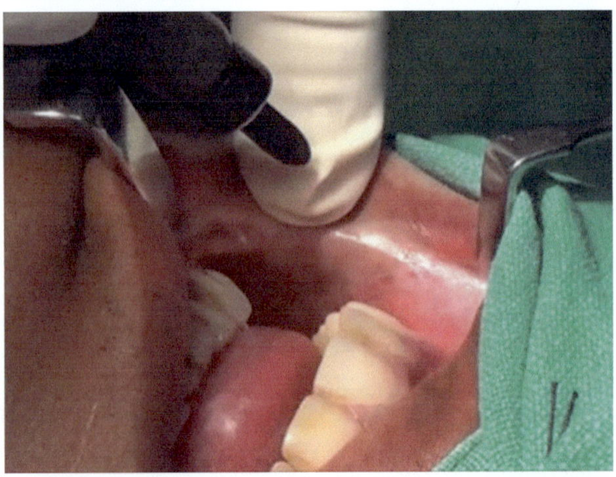

Fig. 4.2 Anterior band

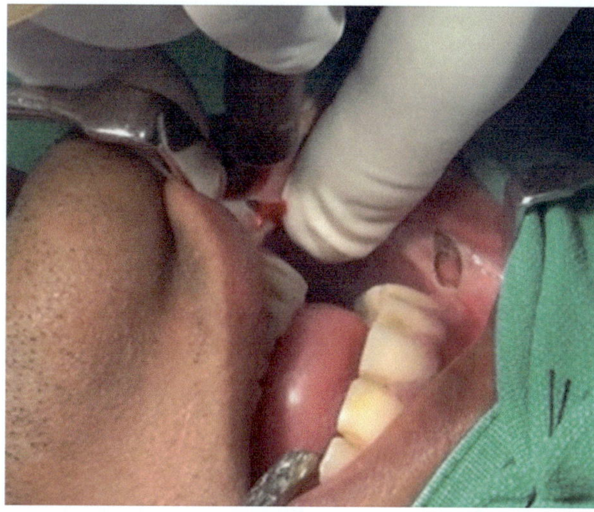

Fig. 4.3 Anterior bands release with Laser

This band extends circumorally from upper sulcus to the lower sulcus, at the level of first premolars. There is a small vessel in the lower part of the cheek band, which needs to be cauterized with bipolar cautery. Doing it in a staggered fashion will facilitate healing. Doing it on both sides in tandem helps intraoral instrumentation. Adequate precaution is to be taken to avoid tearing the commissure muscle.

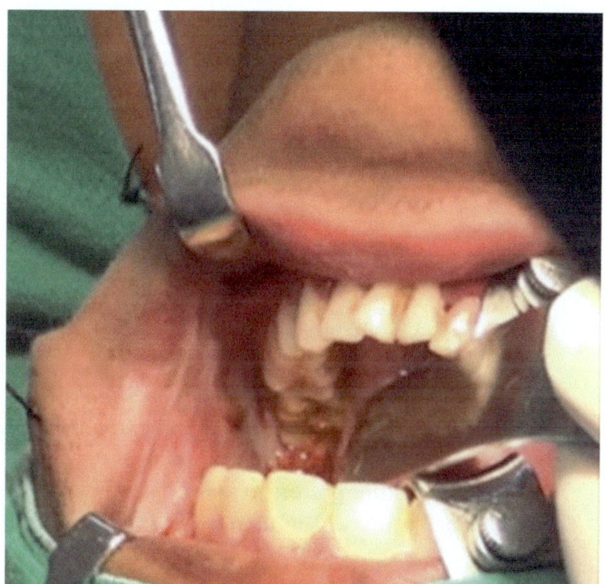

Fig. 4.4 Posterior bands

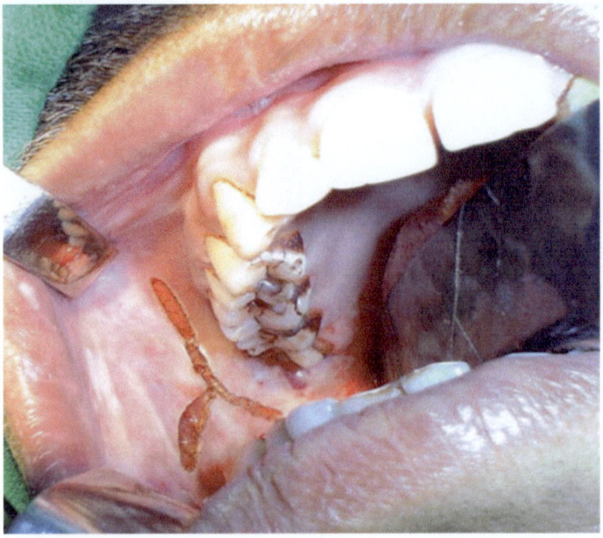

Fig. 4.5 Posterior band release with Laser

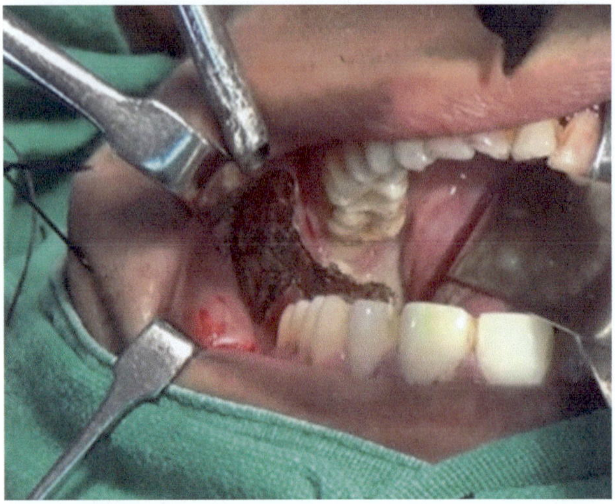

Fig. 4.6 Posterior band release with Laser

These cuts can be fashioned in two ways:

1. Side on Y, which runs few millimeters behind the initial cut and joins at the level of anterior border of the coronoid and extends backward toward the retromolar trigone.
2. Alternatively, author prefers to make a large vertical cut extending over the entire height of the coronoid and then going back toward the retromolar trigone like a T on side.

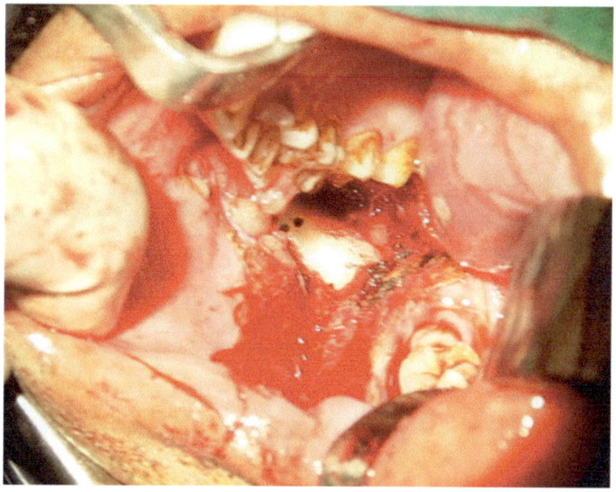

Fig. 4.7 Exposure of coronoid process for coronoidectomy

Release the pterygoid muscles and masseter along the anterior border of the ramus. Need meticulous care of staying subperiosteal on the mandible. The advantage of the bloodless plane ere is soon lost, if we wander into the muscle plains. We cannot overemphasize the need to do both sides in tandem. This release will allow us to ride over the apex of the coronoid process and release the temporalis from its insertion on the coronoid. Retrieval of coronoid after coronoidectomy is facilitated by this complete baring of the coronoid process.

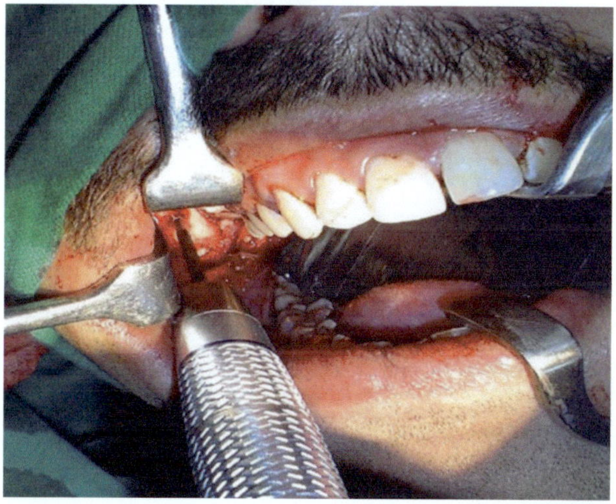

Fig. 4.8 Use of burr for coronoidectomy

The next step is to excise the coronoid process, which is achieved by weakening it by fissure burr and then using osteotome and mallet. Should there be any posterior fibers of temporalis muscle still attached to the coronoid process, the fractures process will get pulled up and lost in the infratemporal fossa. No attempt should be made to retrieve such a coronoid process.

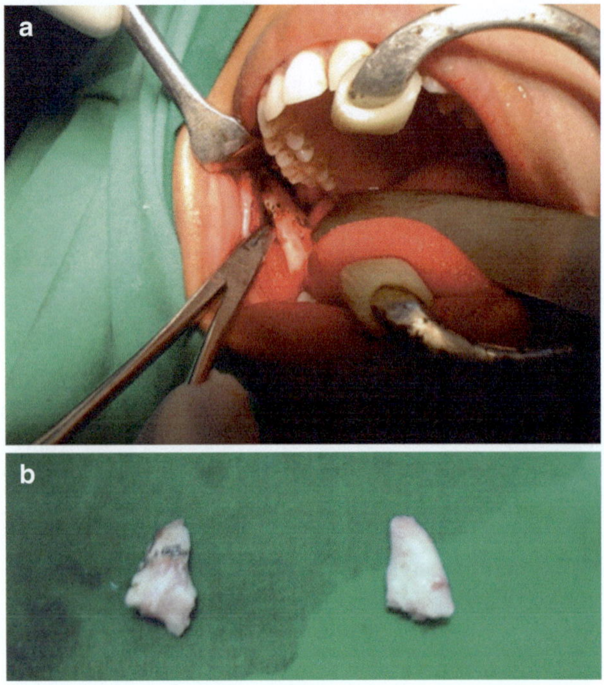

Fig. 4.9 (**a**, **b**) Excision of coronoid processes

Extraction of all last molars is strongly recommended, even if they are healthy. This gives extra space to reconstruct the retromolar trigone and cover the exposed coronoid and ramus.

Coronoidectomy

5

Madan Kapre and Sudhanshu Kothe

Key Points

- Coronoidectomy is the excision of coronoid processes of mandible.
- It is an essential part of release in grades 3 and 4 of trismus.
- Coronoidectomy can be performed with an osteotome, burr, or laser.

We strongly recommend coronoidectomy, as this dramatically improves the results. We have regretted not having done this in our earlier series. Some authors believe in doing high coronoidectomy against radical excision of coronoid. Our philosophy is to get rid of the strong pull of the temporalis muscle, which is the reason for coronoidectomy.

M. Kapre, F.R.C.S., D.L.O. (✉)
Neeti Clinics, Neeti Gaurav Complex, Central Bazar Road, Ramdaspeth,
Nagpur, Maharashtra, India
e-mail: madankapre@gmail.com

S. Kothe, M.S., M.Ch., D.N.B.
Department of Plastic and Reconstructive Surgery, Jai Clinics and Neeti Clinics,
Nagpur, Maharashtra, India
e-mail: sudhanshu.kothe@gmail.com

M. Kapre, S. Kothe (eds.), *Surgery of Trismus in Oral Submucous Fibrosis*,
https://doi.org/10.1007/978-981-10-4892-0_5

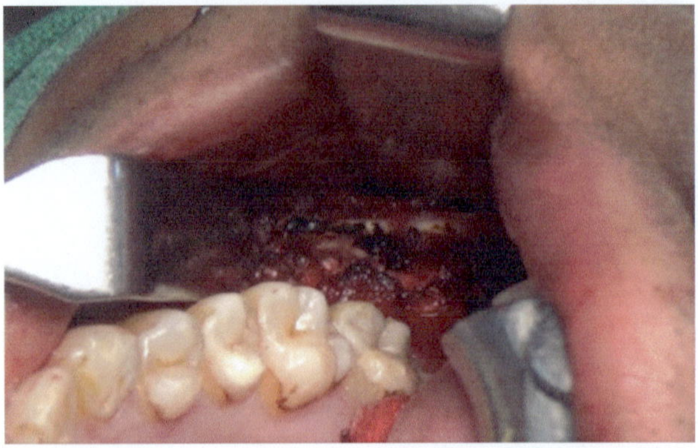

Fig. 5.1 Exposed coronoid process of mandible

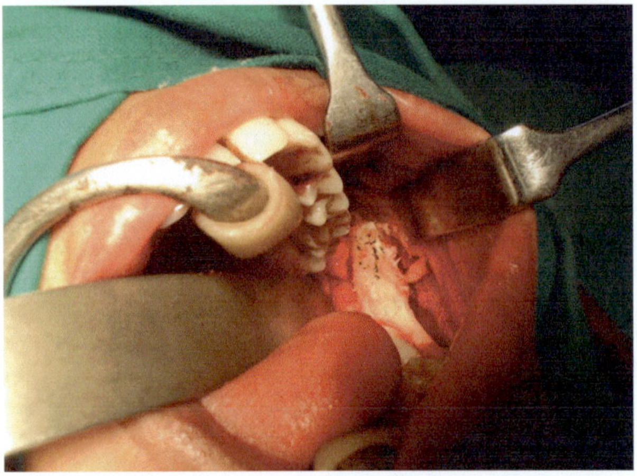

Fig. 5.2 Coronoidectomy procedure

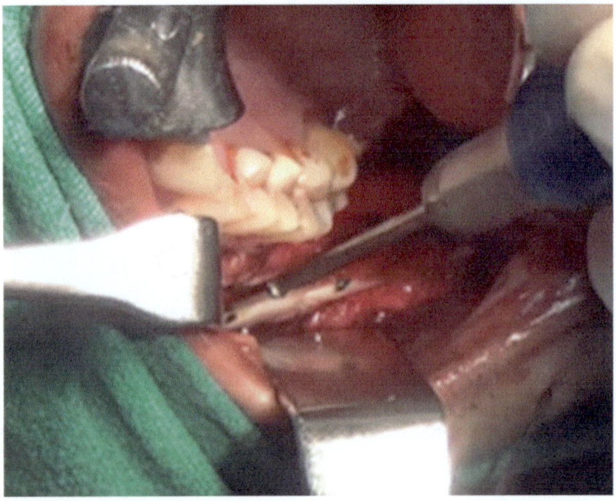

Fig. 5.3 Coronoidectomy with burr

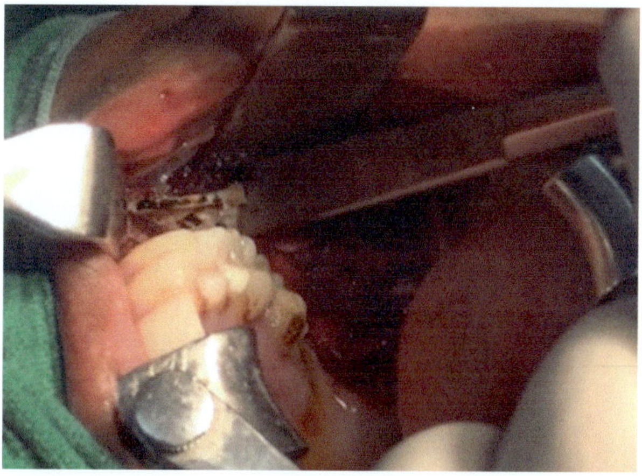

Fig. 5.4 Coronoidectomy with osteotome

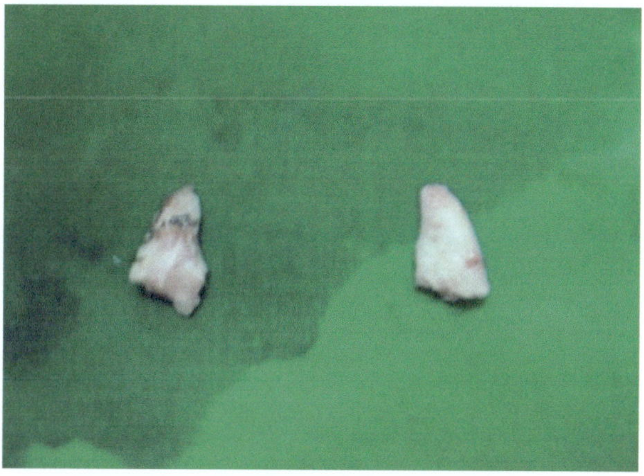

Fig. 5.5 The excised coronoid processes of mandible, after coronoidectomy

Philosophy of Reconstruction

6

Sudhanshu Kothe and Ananya Kothe

Key Points

- Reconstruction is best done with vascularized flaps from intraoral or extra-oral sources.
- Provision of an adequate flap facilitates an adequate release/excision.
- Reconstruction is planned as per the grades of trismus.
- Intraoperative teeth removal facilitates release as well as reconstruction.

After release or excision of affected cheek and surrounding tissues in a case of trismus, there is a need to replace mucosa. Leaving the defects raw will lead to intense fibrosis, with recurrence of trismus.

Replacing the mucosa can be done with many available tissues in and around the mouth.

Skin grafts, split thickness or full thickness, are discouraged, as they will still allow the base of the defect to contract, causing recurrence. Maintaining a skin graft inside the mouth is also fraught with problems.

Alloplastic material is not preferred, as it will not stall the process of intense scarring and recurrence. Any material, be it collagen sheet, will only mimic the epithelium for a short period of a few days and will not be of any further use.

S. Kothe, M.S., M.Ch., D.N.B. (✉)
Department of Plastic and Reconstructive Surgery, Jai Clinics and Neeti Clinics, Nagpur, Maharashtra, India
e-mail: sudhanshu.kothe@gmail.com

A. Kothe, B.D.S.
24, Gajanan Nagar, Wardha Road, Nagpur 440015, Maharashtra, India
e-mail: ananya.kothe@gmail.com

M. Kapre, S. Kothe (eds.), *Surgery of Trismus in Oral Submucous Fibrosis*,
https://doi.org/10.1007/978-981-10-4892-0_6

Reconstruction can be done with intraoral tissues of tissues from the extraoral sources. Intraoral choices are mucosal flaps like mandibular mucoperiosteal flap or palatal mucoperiosteal flaps. It could also be a musculomucosal flap like the tongue flap. Flaps bring in their own blood supply and thus vascularize the bed of the defect in submucous fibrosis. Muscle flaps further enhance the vascularity of the area.

Extraoral source is the platysma flap and its variations. These flaps are sturdy, pliable, and well vascularized. They give epithelial lining to the defect and also create many planes of movement within the cheek, for supple movements. The platysma myocutaneous flap has areolar layers between the skin and muscle and the muscle and fascia under it; hence, once the flap is inset, the tissues can move between themselves to give a supple cheek.

Choice of reconstruction is dictated by the site and area of defect in the cheeks, which in turn is dictated by the grade of trismus. In grade 1 and 2, the defect may be only a linear cut, of a small defect in the posterior cheek, in the retromolar area. Reconstruction, if necessary, could be in the form of mucosal flaps or tongue flap. In grade 3 trismus, often, the defect is large and involves the posterior and mid-cheek, along with an exposed mandible due to coronoidectomy. Here, larger flaps, like the palatal flap, may be necessary. In grade 4 trismus, the entire mucosa of the cheek, and may be the palate to some extent, will be lost, and the mandible is exposed due to coronoidectomy. Here, platysma myocutaneous flap is the preferred option.

An important prerequisite for good result is an adequate release. If the surgeon releasing and excising the fibrotic tissues is assured that the defects can be covered well, using adequate flaps, there is better likelihood of adequate release. This is how a good reconstruction positively influences a good release and result.

Managing the Teeth

Managing teeth is an important aspect of trismus. Oral hygiene is paramount.

During release, often, the last teeth, i.e., third or second molars, may have to be extracted, to create more space posteriorly and to also facilitate reconstruction. To transpose the mandibular mucoperiosteal flap, the third molar of the mandible is removed, so as to move the flap into the retromolar area and avoid a fold formation there. The third molar may also land up biting the flap, if it is not extracted. Palatal flap transposition requires removal of maxillary third molars, as these teeth are likely to get buried behind the flap pedicle. The bony ridge around the third molars is also ground down, or nibbled off, to facilitate transposition of palatal flap.

Platysma flap skin mucosalizes fairly well. It may take 1–2 years for that to occur.

In some instances, flaps had to be trimmed, to avoid bite injuries to the flaps.

7 The Fat Flap

Madan Kapre, Harsh Karan Gupta, and Sudhanshu Kothe

Key Points
- The fat flap is derived from buccal pad of fat.
- The cheek epithelializes by secondary intention.

The disadvantages are that these flaps are random pattern and may not have adequate blood supply. They may necrose often and lead to fibrosis and recurrence of trismus. They do not have epithelium and hence heal by secondary intention.

M. Kapre, F.R.C.S., D.L.O. (✉) • H.K. Gupta, M.S., D.N.B. (ENT)
Neeti Clinics, Neeti Gaurav Complex, Central Bazar Road, Ramdaspeth,
Nagpur, Maharashtra, India
e-mail: madankapre@gmail.com; harshkarangupta@gmail.com

S. Kothe, M.S., M.Ch., D.N.B.
Department of Plastic and Reconstructive Surgery, Jai Clinics and Neeti Clinics,
Nagpur, Maharashtra, India
e-mail: sudhanshu.kothe@gmail.com

M. Kapre, S. Kothe (eds.), *Surgery of Trismus in Oral Submucous Fibrosis*,
https://doi.org/10.1007/978-981-10-4892-0_7

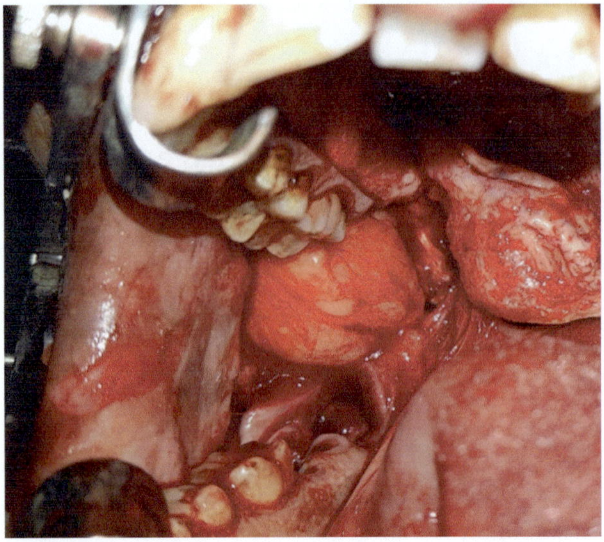

Fig. 7.1 The fat flap is a flap of buccal fat, raised from the defect itself. It is a random pattern flap

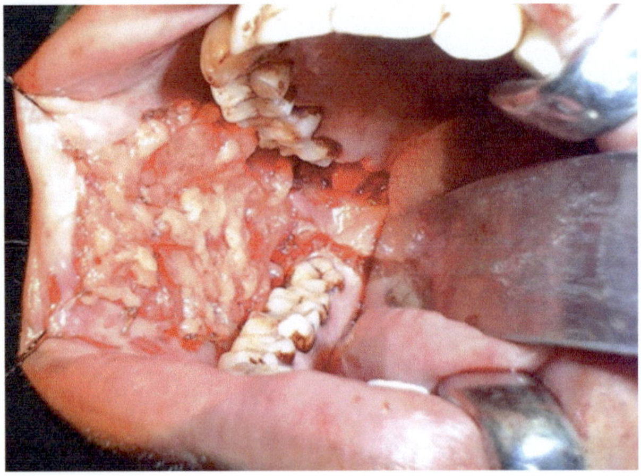

Fig. 7.2 The fat is eventually expected to epithelialize, and the wound heals by secondary intention

8 Nasolabial Flaps

Madan Kapre, Abhishek Vaidya, and Sudhanshu Kothe

Key Points

- These are thin flaps from the cheek.
- They leave behind unsightly scars on the face.
- The width of nasolabial flap does not cover the cheek defects in grade 4 trismus.

The nasolabial flaps are skin and subcutaneous tissue flaps from the nasolabial area. They are superiorly based and are tunneled through a gap into the cheek and delivered into the mouth.

Advantages are that they are reliable and local.

Disadvantages are that they are small in size. They are inadequate for defects of the entire cheek, as may be found after release for grade 4 trismus or grade 3 trismus. They leave unsightly scars in the visible area of the cheek.

M. Kapre, F.R.C.S., D.L.O. (✉) • A. Vaidya, M.S., D.N.B. (ENT)
Neeti Clinics, Neeti Gaurav Complex, Central Bazar Road, Ramdaspeth, Nagpur, Maharashtra, India
e-mail: madankapre@gmail.com; abhishek.d.vaidya@gmail.com

S. Kothe, M.S., M.Ch., D.N.B.
Department of Plastic and Reconstructive Surgery, Jai Clinics and Neeti Clinics, Nagpur, Maharashtra, India
e-mail: sudhanshu.kothe@gmail.com

M. Kapre, S. Kothe (eds.), *Surgery of Trismus in Oral Submucous Fibrosis*,
https://doi.org/10.1007/978-981-10-4892-0_8

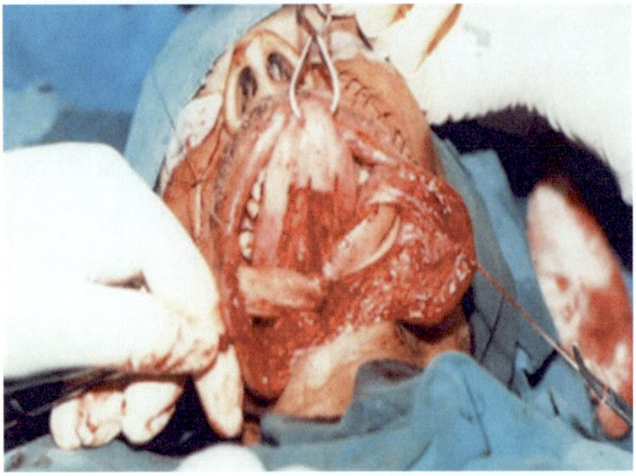

Fig. 8.1 Nasolabial flaps

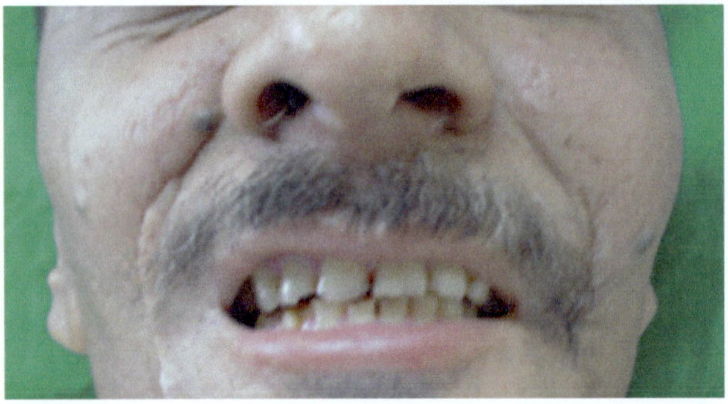

Fig. 8.2 Facial scars following nasolabial flaps

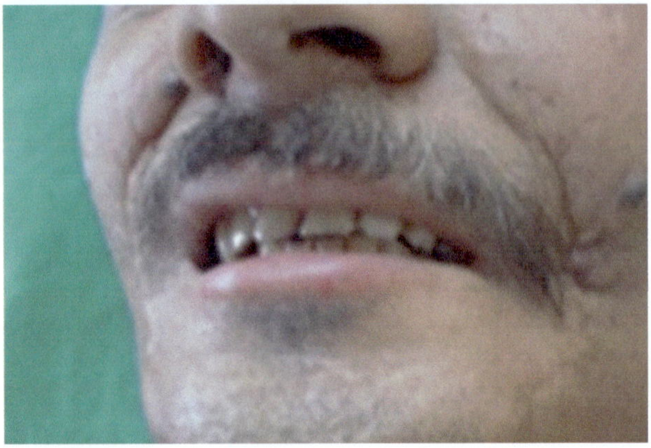

Fig. 8.3 Facial scars following nasolabial flaps

The Tongue Flap

9

Sudhanshu Kothe

Key Points
- These flaps are raised from the tongue.
- They may be based anteriorly or posteriorly.
- Size is a limitation.

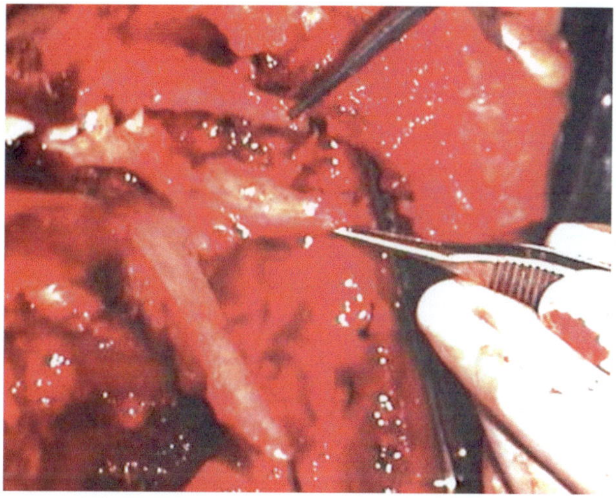

Fig. 9.1 Tongue flaps

S. Kothe, M.S., M.Ch., D.N.B.
Department of Plastic and Reconstructive Surgery, Jai Clinics and Neeti Clinics, Nagpur, Maharashtra, India
e-mail: sudhanshu.kothe@gmail.com

M. Kapre, S. Kothe (eds.), *Surgery of Trismus in Oral Submucous Fibrosis*,
https://doi.org/10.1007/978-981-10-4892-0_9

We do not use tongue flap as a primary measure anymore. It may be used in grade 2 or grade 3 trismus, where the defect is in the posterior cheek. A lateral posteriorly based flap of the tongue is harvested and rotated into the defect in the retromolar area. It may not be very long.

The flap is sturdy, and vascular, and available near the defect itself, i.e., retromolar area.

The disadvantage is that there is a fold formation behind the flap, and tethering of the tongue may occur, with obliteration of the lateral floor of the mouth.

If such a fold occurs, it is recommended that the flap be divided, the fold obliterated, and the tongue be freed secondarily, once the patient maintains good mouth opening.

The Mandibular Mucoperiosteal Flap 10

Madan Kapre and Sudhanshu Kothe

Key Points

- Mandibular mucoperiosteal flap (MMPF) is a mucosal flap from the medial aspect of the mandible.
- It is a reliable random pattern flap of native mucosa.
- Useful for covering small posterior defects in the cheek, especially exposed mandible after coronoidectomy.

Limitation of this flap is the size. But in cases where the mucosal defect is small, and the mandible is exposed, especially after coronoidectomy, this flap is useful.

M. Kapre, F.R.C.S., D.L.O. (✉)
Neeti Clinics, Neeti Gaurav Complex, Central Bazar Road, Ramdaspeth, Nagpur, Maharashtra, India
e-mail: madankapre@gmail.com

S. Kothe, M.S., M.Ch., D.N.B.
Department of Plastic and Reconstructive Surgery, Jai Clinics and Neeti Clinics, Nagpur, Maharashtra, India
e-mail: sudhanshu.kothe@gmail.com

M. Kapre, S. Kothe (eds.), *Surgery of Trismus in Oral Submucous Fibrosis*,
https://doi.org/10.1007/978-981-10-4892-0_10

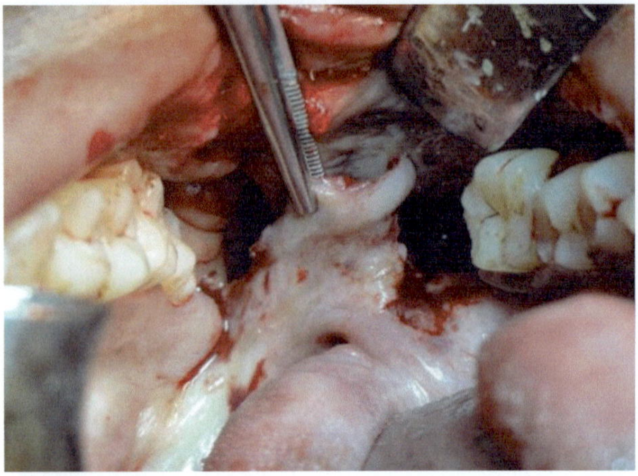

Fig. 10.1 This flap is elevated from the area of mucosa over the lingual surface of the mandible, based posteriorly

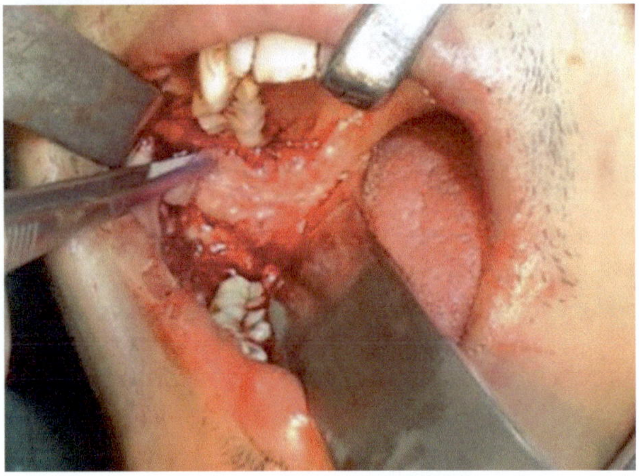

Fig. 10.2 Lateral floor of the mouth and lateral inferior mucosa over the tongue are usually included in the flap

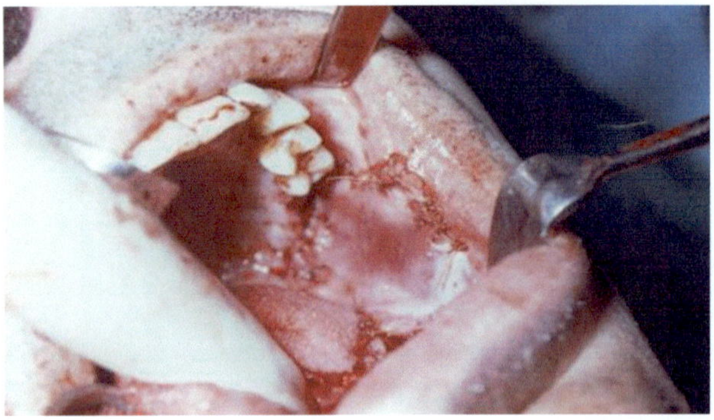

Fig. 10.3 A strip of length 5 cm and width 2.5 cm can be harvested as a flap, to cover defects in the retromolar area. Hence, it is useful for grade 1, 2, and 3 trismus

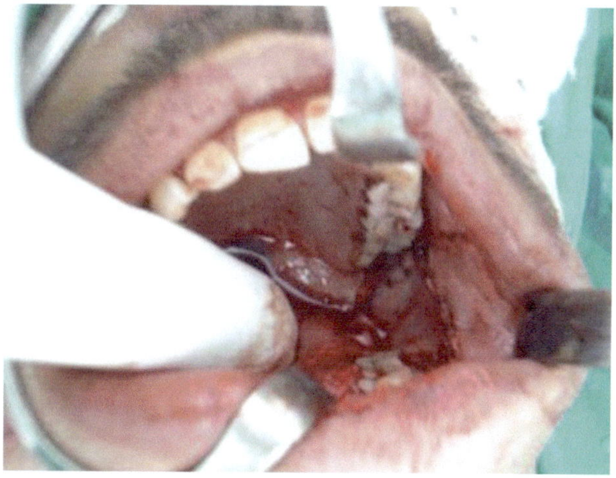

Fig. 10.4 Previously, we were using larger flaps but now restrict ourselves to smaller flaps, as they are more reliable

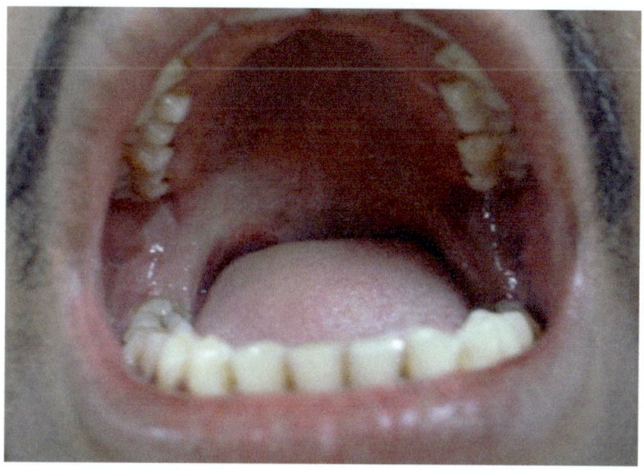

Fig. 10.5 Postoperative photograph. The outline of the flap cannot be made out easily

The Palatal Flap

11

Sudhanshu Kothe

Key Points

- Palatal mucoperiosteal flaps are sturdy axial pattern flaps based on greater palatine artery.
- Full hard palate flap can be used for unilateral cheek or hemipalatal flaps for bilateral defects.
- Donor area heals well, within 4 weeks.

The palatal flap is an important source of tissue for reconstruction. It is useful in grade 2, 3, and sometimes grade 4 trismus patients.

Whole palatal mucoperiosteal flap from the hard palate area can be elevated on the greater palatine artery pedicle. The palate can be used for covering bilateral defects by dividing in the midline and elevating two flaps on each side or unilateral cover based on a single side artery.

It is a sturdy flap, with good axial blood supply. Preserving a small mucoperiosteal bridge posteriorly, behind the pedicle, can enhance the venous drainage of the flap, to improve the survival of the flap.

Palatal mucoperiosteal flap incision along the edges of the hard palate and few millimeters anterior to the posterior edge of the hard palate.

S. Kothe, M.S., M.Ch., D.N.B.
Department of Plastic and Reconstructive Surgery, Jai Clinics and Neeti Clinics, Nagpur, Maharashtra, India
e-mail: sudhanshu.kothe@gmail.com

M. Kapre, S. Kothe (eds.), *Surgery of Trismus in Oral Submucous Fibrosis*,
https://doi.org/10.1007/978-981-10-4892-0_11

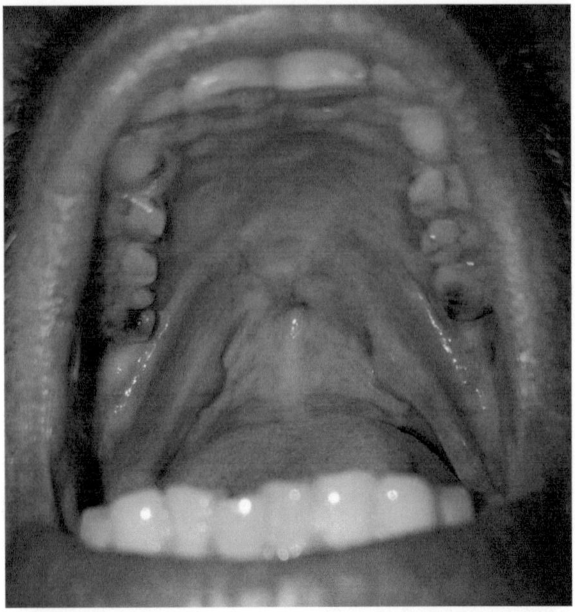

Fig. 11.1 Result after bilateral Palatal flap reconstruction: Anterior view

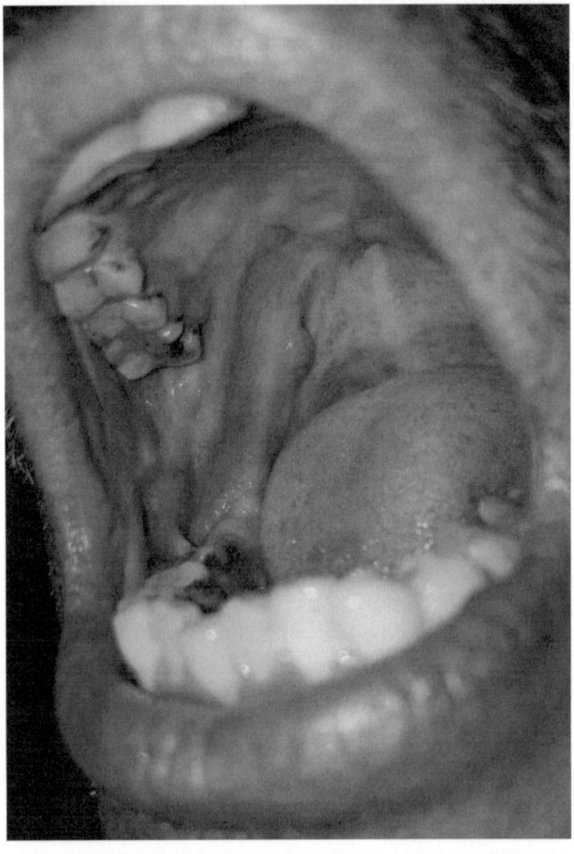

Fig. 11.2 Result after palatal flap reconstruction

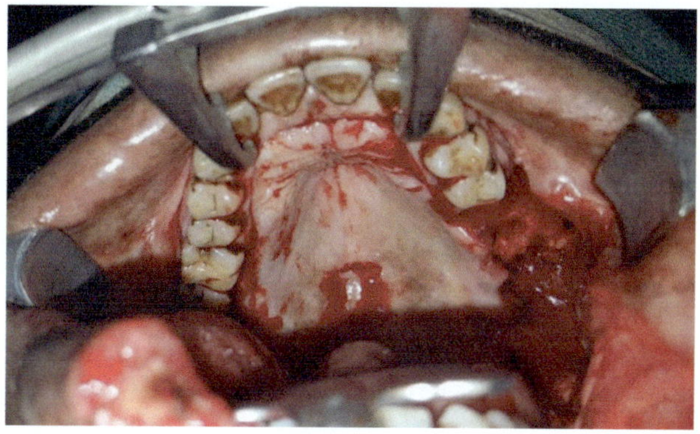

Fig. 11.3 Technique of raising palatal flap: Incision

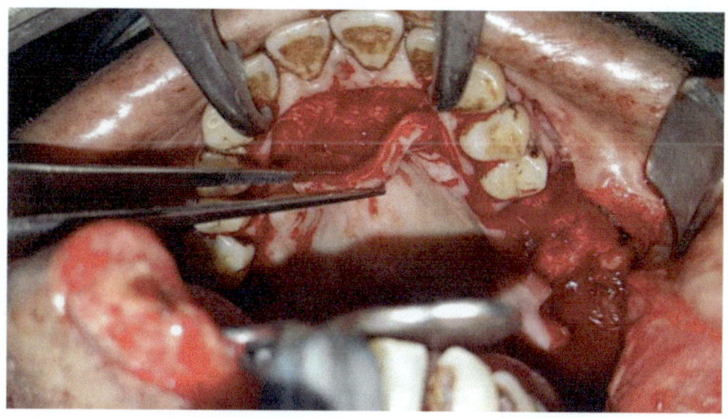

Fig. 11.4 Raising the flap, starting anteriorly

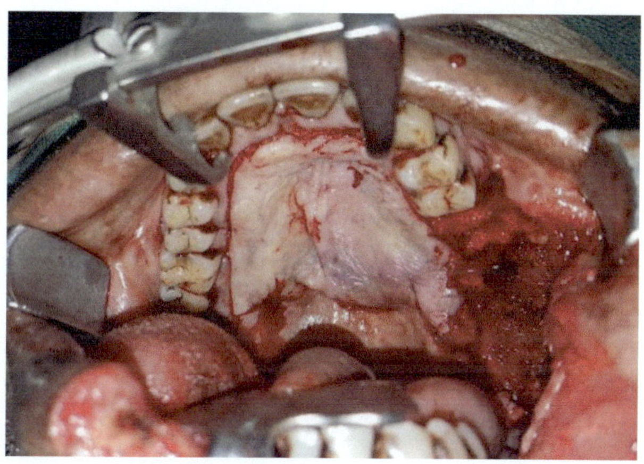

Fig. 11.5 The raised flap based on the left side pedicle

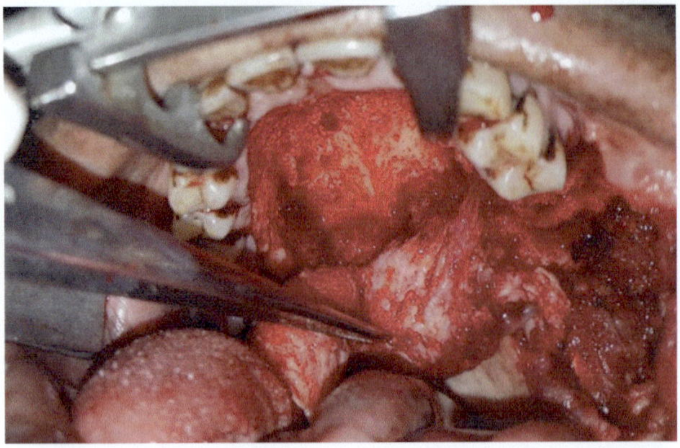

Fig. 11.6 Flap based on the left greater palatine pedicle

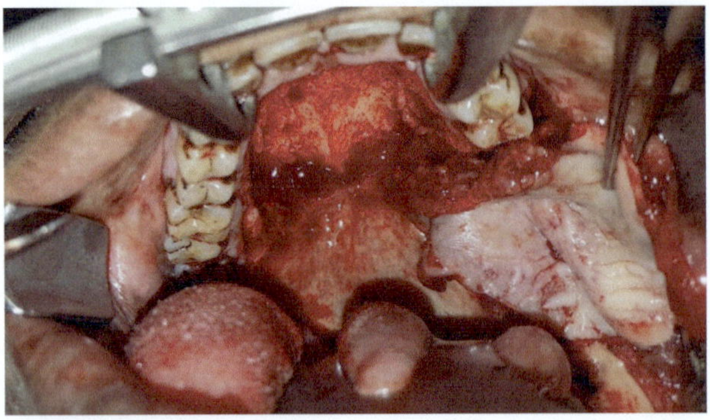

Fig. 11.7 Flap rotated into the left cheek

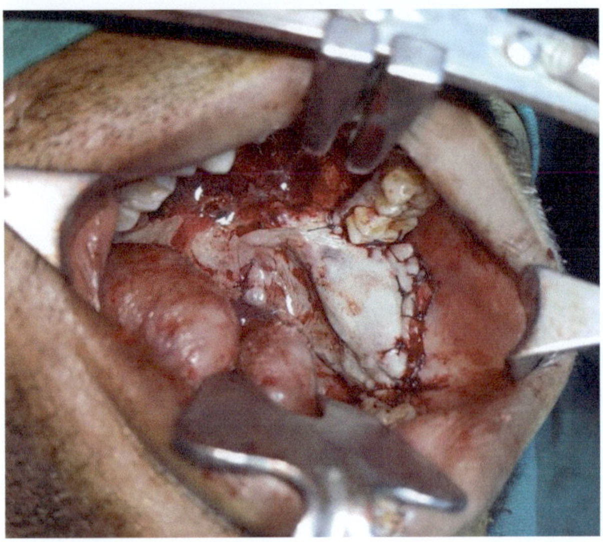

Fig. 11.8 Palatal flap inset, intraoperative view, for a retromolar defect for grade 3 trismus

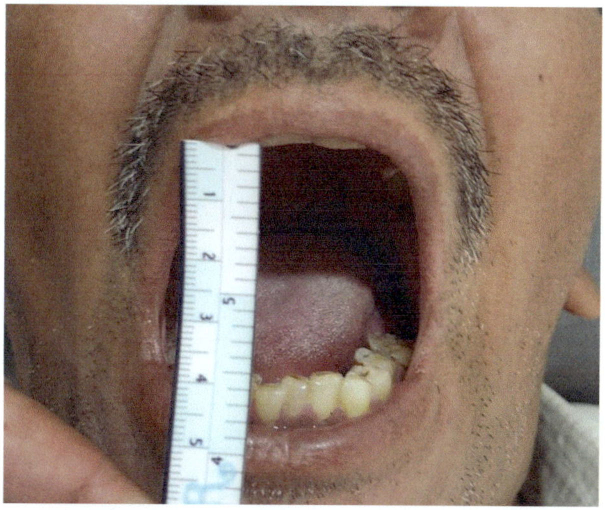

Fig. 11.9 Mouth opening after trismus release and bilateral hemipalatal flap

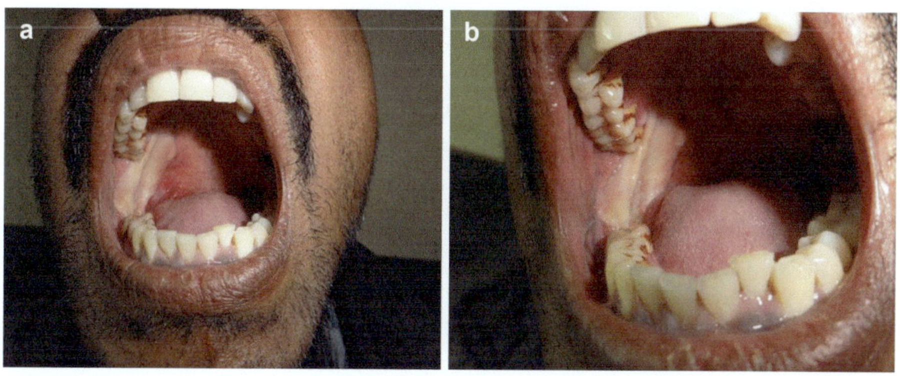

Fig. 11.10 (**a**, **b**) Whole palate unilaterally based flaps can cover almost the entire cheek, barring the area of the commissure

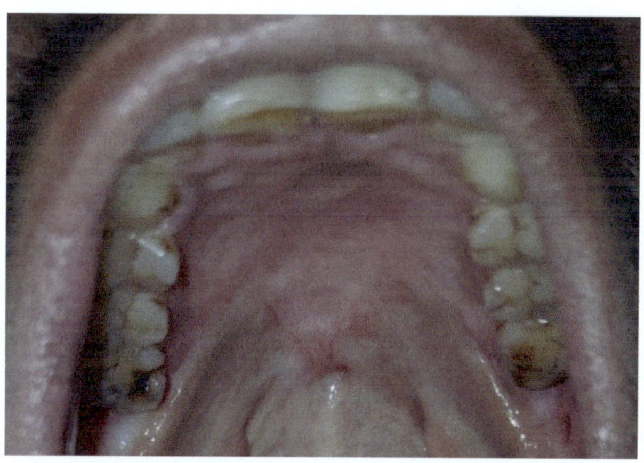

Fig. 11.11 The healed hard palate donor area

The Platysma Myocutaneous Flap

12

Sudhanshu Kothe

Key Points

- A reliable regional flap based on perforators. Uses tissues unaffected by OSMF.
- Useful for grade 4 trismus, in defects involving large areas of cheek lining and adjoining areas like the palate posteriorly and lower lip anteriorly.
- Large area of the skin from the inferior part of the neck can be harvested for defects of the cheek.

Platysma myocutaneous flap is a flap of the skin and muscle, raised from the lower neck, based on the platysma muscle, superiorly. The blood supply of the flap comes from the mental branch of the facial artery, in the submental region.

The flap is raised from below upward, including the deep cervical fascia over the sternomastoid muscle and including the external jugular vein.

The flap is tunneled through the subcutaneous plane over the mandible, into the cheek. Large defects involving the entire cheek mucosa can be covered with this flap. Hence, it is used in grade 4 trismus. The flap can reach and cover soft palate posteriorly, to lower lip anteriorly.

S. Kothe, M.S., M.Ch., D.N.B.
Department of Plastic and Reconstructive Surgery, Jai Clinics and Neeti Clinics, Nagpur, Maharashtra, India
e-mail: sudhanshu.kothe@gmail.com

M. Kapre, S. Kothe (eds.), *Surgery of Trismus in Oral Submucous Fibrosis*,
https://doi.org/10.1007/978-981-10-4892-0_12

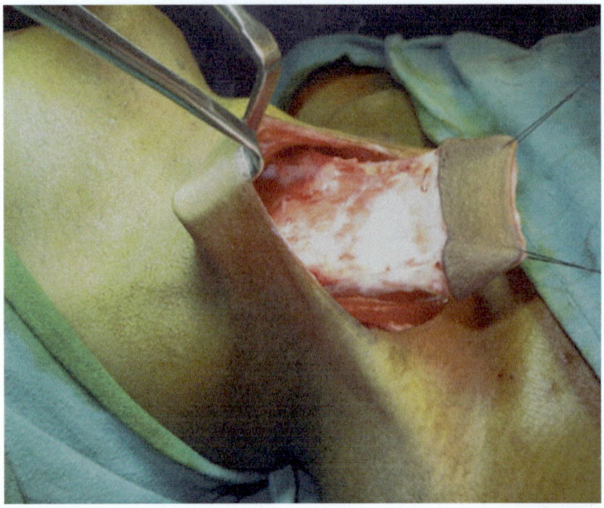

Fig. 12.1 The raised Platysma myocutaneous flap

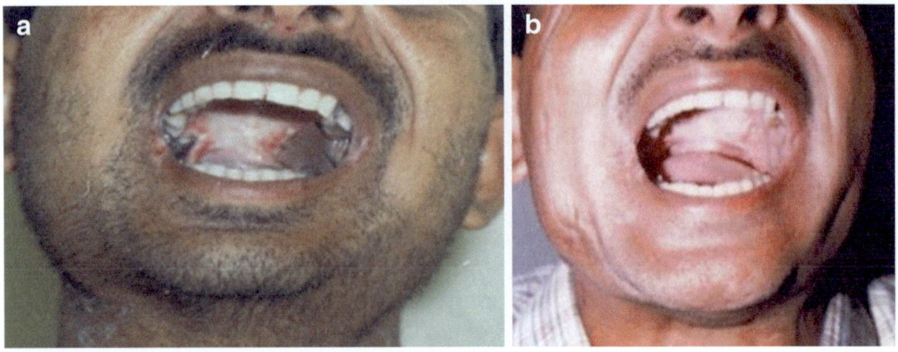

Fig. 12.2 (**a**, **b**) Early and late results of Platysma myocutaneous flaps

The skin of the flap mucosalizes over a period of 1–2 years.

As it settles in the mouth, there is apparent increase in its size and dimensions, leading to further improvement in the mouth opening of the patient.

Above picture shows mouth opening after 3 weeks of surgery on the left and 13 months postoperative on the right.

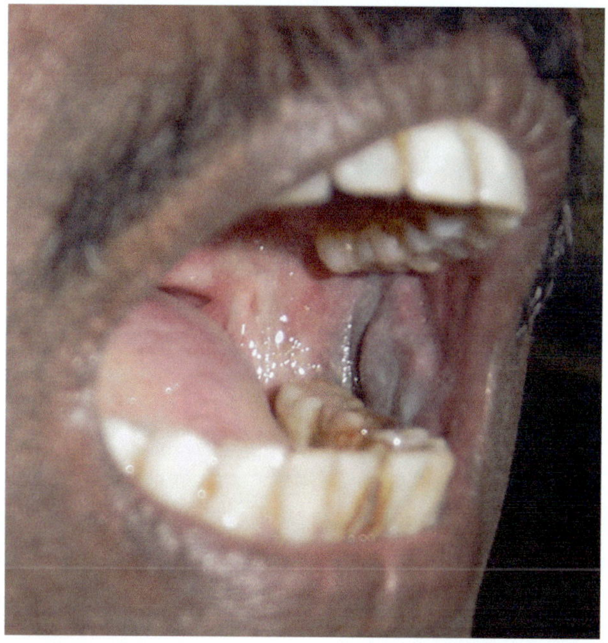

Fig. 12.3 Mucosalization of the skin of platysma myocutaneous flap, 1 year postoperative. Result of a grade 4 trismus

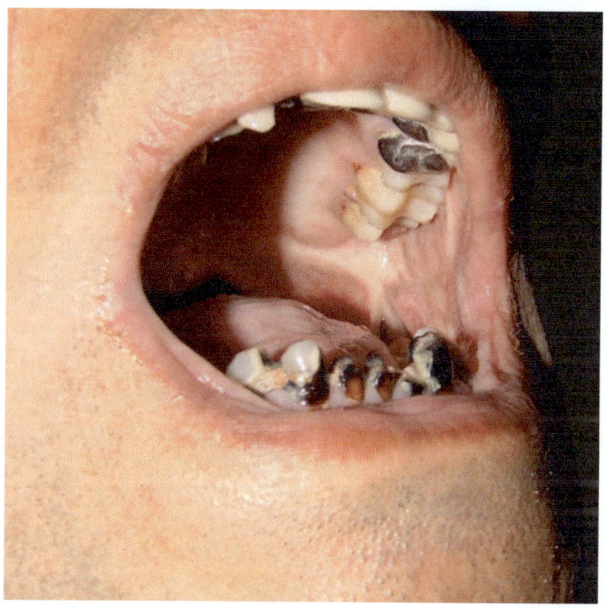

Fig. 12.4 Mucosalization of the skin of platysma myocutaneous flap, 9 years postoperative. Result of a grade 4 trismus who had 0 mm mouth-opening preoperatively

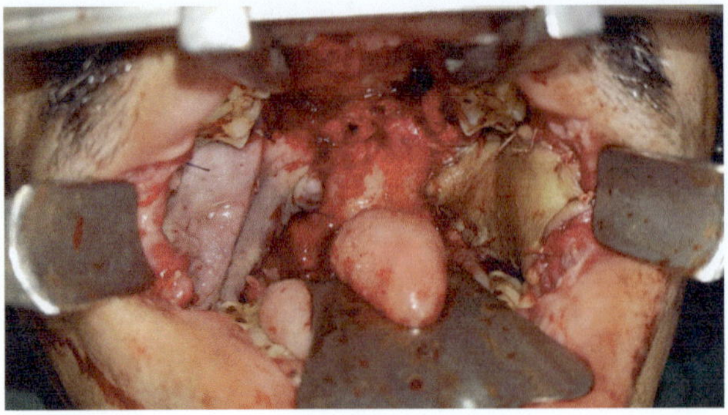

Fig. 12.5 Bilateral reconstruction: right side palatal mucoperiosteal flap, left side platysma myocutaneous flap

Technique

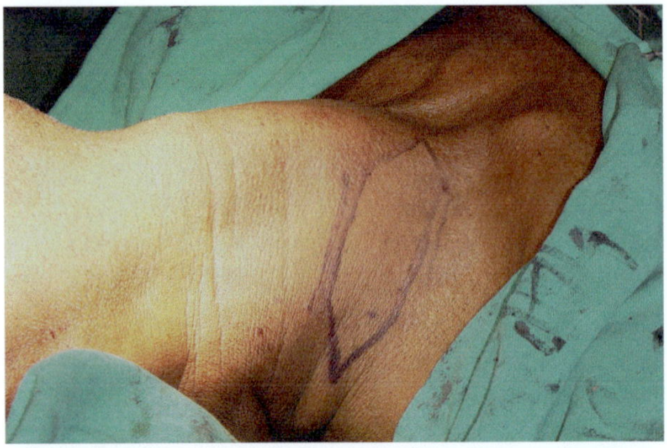

Fig. 12.6 Skin markings

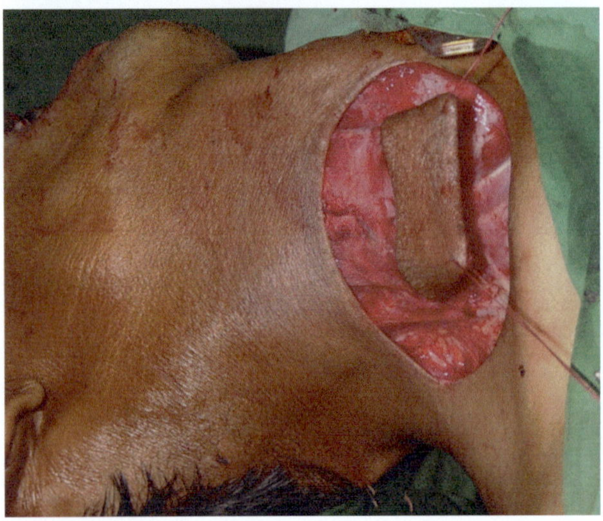

Fig. 12.7 Raising of flap

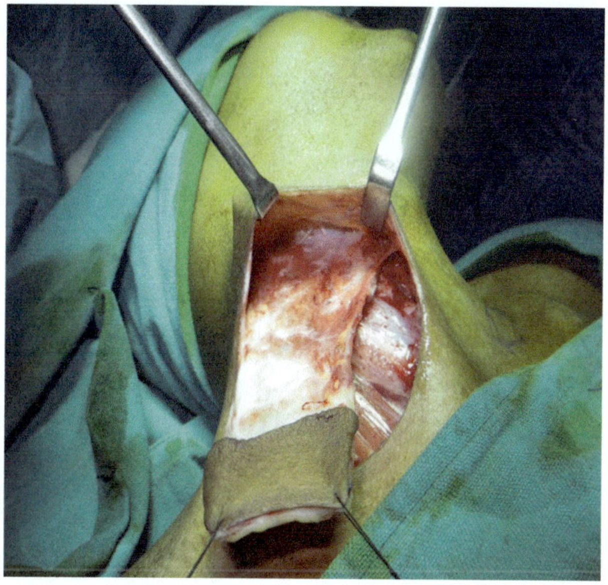

Fig. 12.8 The raised platysma myocutaneous flap

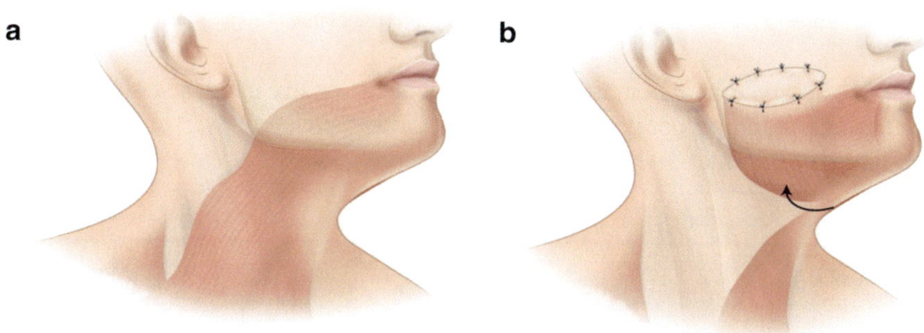

Fig. 12.9 (**a**, **b**) The flap is passed over the mandible subcutaneously and delivered into the intraoral cheek defect

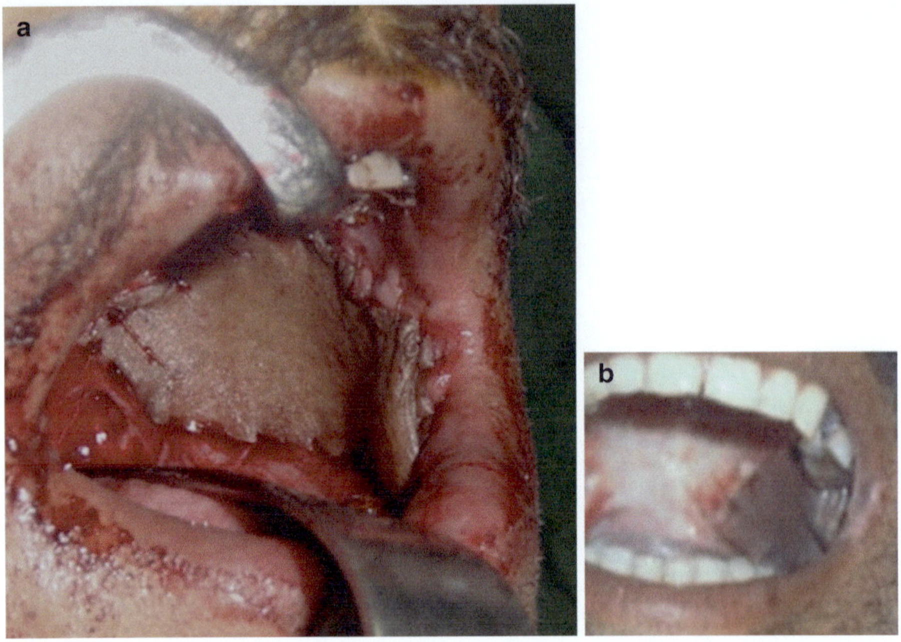

Fig. 12.10 (**a**, **b**) Platysma myocutaneous flap inset into the cheek defect

The skin of platysma myocutaneous flap may occasionally undergo color changes. The flap may undergo congestion and look darker between day 2 and day 4. The color returns to normal in the latter half of the week.

Fig. 12.11 Platysma myocutaneous flap on day 1

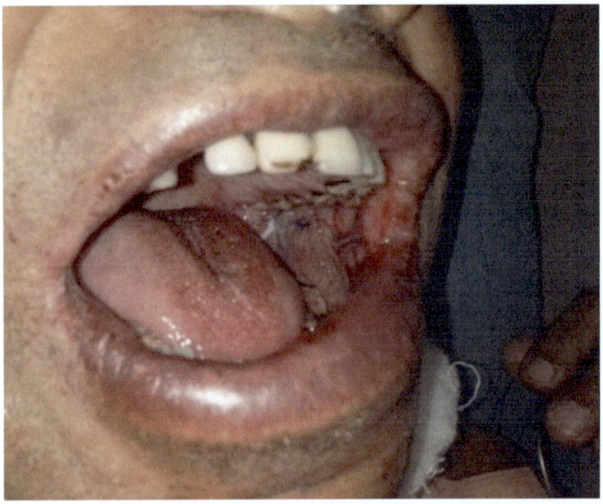

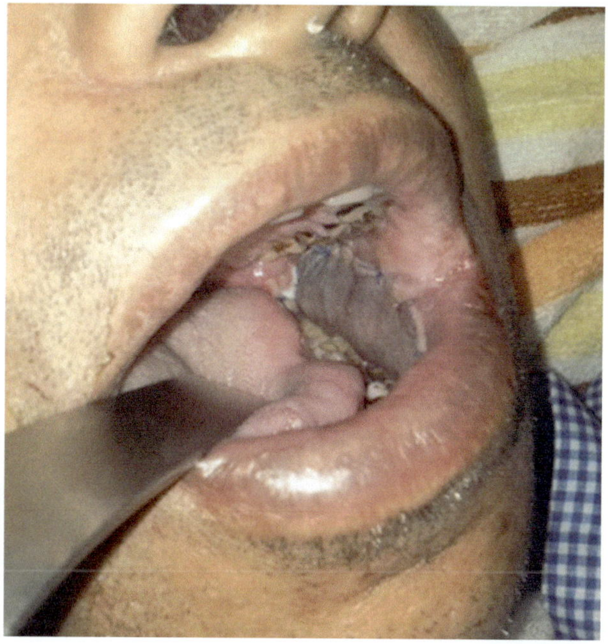

Fig. 12.12 The flap on day 2—congestive changes

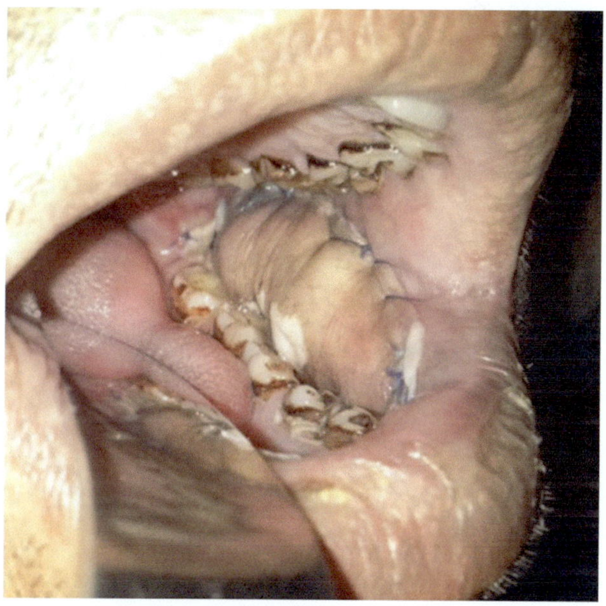

Fig. 12.13 The flap on day 4—congestive relieved, flap healthy

These congestive changes have reduced in incidence after we started including the external jugular vein in the flap while raising.

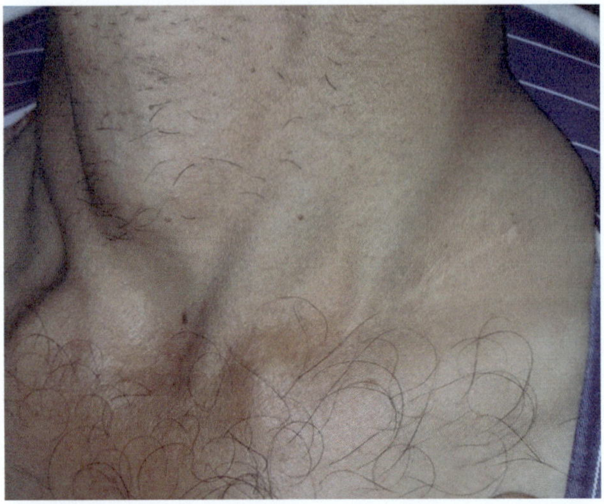

Fig. 12.14 The donor area neck following platysma myocutaneous flap

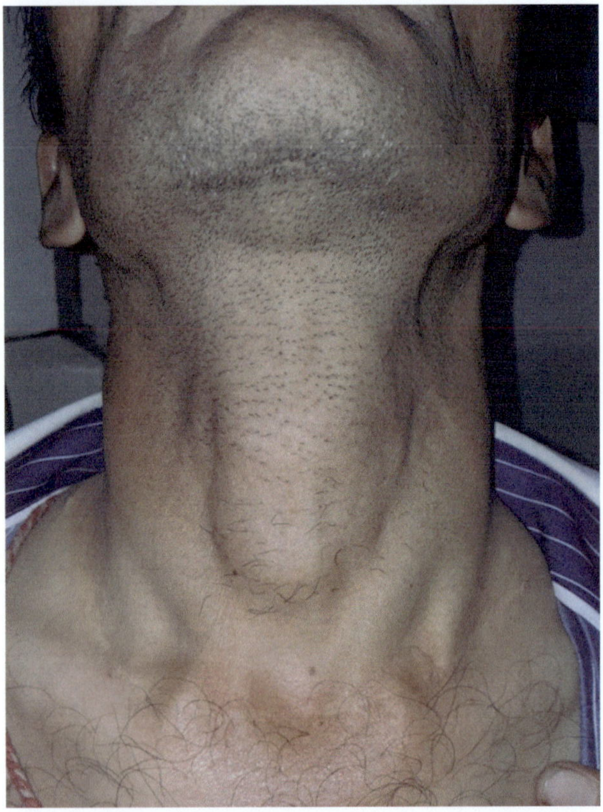

Fig. 12.15 The appearance of the neck and scars in the neck following platysma myocutaneous flap. The scars are barely visible

The Platysma Myofascial Flap

13

Sudhanshu Kothe

Key Points

- Platysma-based axial pattern flap, without including the skin.
- Gives sturdy cover to the cheek.
- Epithelialization occurs in 4–8 weeks.

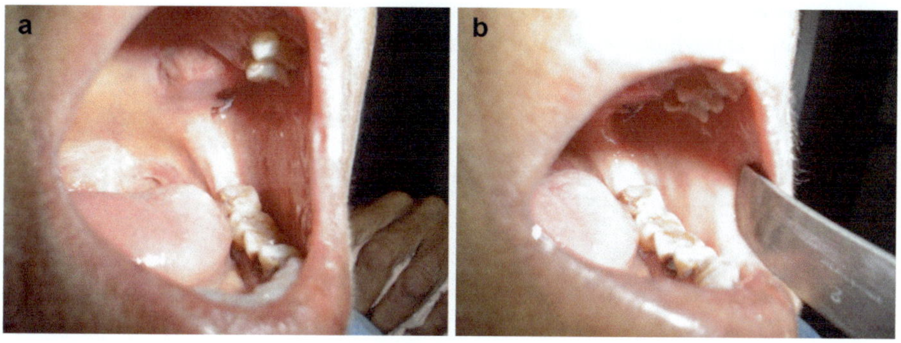

Fig. 13.1 (**a, b**) Healed and epithelialized platysma myofascial flap in the cheek

S. Kothe, M.S., M.Ch., D.N.B.
Department of Plastic and Reconstructive Surgery, Jai Clinics and Neeti Clinics, Nagpur, Maharshtra, India
e-mail: sudhanshu.kothe@gmail.com

M. Kapre, S. Kothe (eds.), *Surgery of Trismus in Oral Submucous Fibrosis*,
https://doi.org/10.1007/978-981-10-4892-0_13

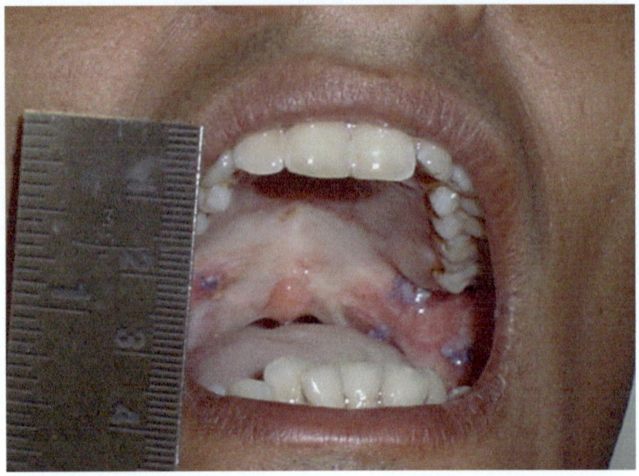

Fig. 13.2 Mouth opening after platysma myofascial flap

In situations where the skin of platysma flap cannot be harvested, a platysma myofascial flap can be elevated, to cover the entire area of mucosa of the cheek. It will epithelialize over a period of 3–8 weeks, to give adequate cover in grade 3 and 4 trismus.

In cases where there is loss of skin in platysma myocutaneous flap due to necrosis, the muscle will survive and work as a myofascial flap, to give adequate cover. In such instances, debridement of the skin of the flap is undertaken with an eye on the surviving muscle, which is left behind, attached to the cheek raw area.

Postoperative Care

14

Vidula Kapre and Gauri Vaidya

Key Points

- Long-term success depends heavily on postoperative care.
- Postoperative pain relief is paramount to management.
- Medications and blocks are useful adjuncts.
- Mouth-opening exercises need counselling and strict follow-up.

More than with any other surgical procedure, in case of surgery for trismus due to OSMF, long-term success depends heavily on good postoperative care.

The inherent nature of the pathology is to induce submucous fibrosis, and once good mouth opening is achieved surgically, we have to strive to maintain it postoperatively avoiding recurrent fibrosis.

The cornerstones in achieving this are:

- Postoperative pain relief
- Good oral hygiene
- Regular and effective mouth-opening exercise

V. Kapre (✉) • G. Vaidya
Neeti Clinics, Neeti Gaurav Complex, Central Bazar Road, Ramdaspeth, Nagpur, Maharashtra, India
e-mail: vidulakapre@gmail.com; gauri.kapre@gmail.com

M. Kapre, S. Kothe (eds.), *Surgery of Trismus in Oral Submucous Fibrosis*,
https://doi.org/10.1007/978-981-10-4892-0_14

Pain Relief

The main hurdle against performing mouth-opening exercises and maintaining oral hygiene is pain. Hence we have a standard pain management protocol by way of nerve block and analgesics.

Systemic analgesics are administered round the clock. Multidrug regime is employed. Combination of nonsteroidal anti-inflammatory drug (NSAID) (e.g. diclofenac) and opioid (e.g. tramadol) is found to be effective.

The protocol for nerve blocks is to administer mandibular nerve blocks with local anaesthetic solution (e.g. Sensorcaine 2 mL of 0.5% solution) along with long-acting steroid depot preparation (1 mL) which is injected on second postoperative day, every alternate day there after till the date of discharge and on follow-up visits at two weekly interval for first 2 months.

The technique for nerve block may be:

Intraoral. Needle is inserted immediately medial to the anterior border of the ramus of mandible, approximately 1 cm above the occlusal surface of the third molar. The syringe is parallel to the occlusal surface of the lower jaw. The needle is advanced along the medial side of ramus to a depth of 2 cm, and simultaneously the syringe is rotated over the premolar region of the opposite side of the mandible. The local anaesthetic and steroid solution is injected.

Extraoral. Needle is inserted 1 cm below and anterior to midpoint of zygomatic process, perpendicular to the skin. The needle is advanced to a depth of 2–3 cm, and the solution of local anaesthetic and steroid is injected.

Vazirani-Akinosi technique is an intraoral technique where the patient is not required to open the mouth. It is a closed-mouth technique wherein the cheek is retracted. Needle is inserted at the reflection of gingival to buccal mucosa parallel to occlusal surface and behind the last molar. The needle is advanced to a depth of 1.5–2 cm staying just medial to the ramous of the mandible. Local anaesthetic and steroid solutions are injected.

Intraoral Technique

Landmark: anterior border of ramus of the mandible or oblique line is located with left index finger.

Injection site: immediately medial to oblique line and 1 cm above the occlusal surface of third molar.

Direction: syringe should lie horizontal, parallel to the body of the mandible and occlusal surface of the lower jaw.

Technique: needle is inserted at the injection site and slowly advanced along the medial side of the ramus to a depth of 2 cm; at the same time, syringe is rotated in the horizontal plane towards premolar region of opposite side of the mandible.

Solution: 2 mL of 0.5 % bupivacaine + 1 mL of Depo-Medrol

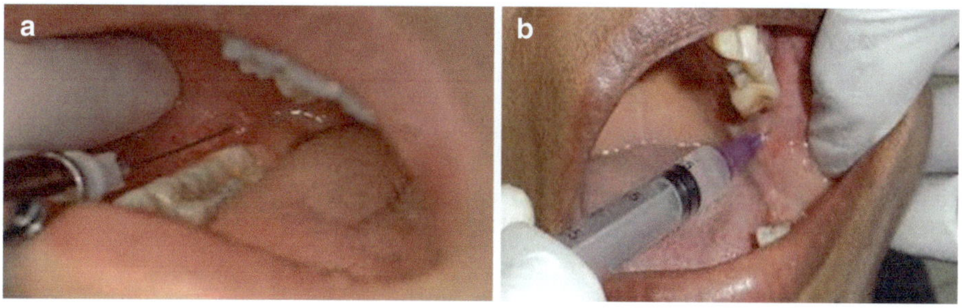

Fig. 14.1 (**a**, **b**) Intraoral technique

Extraoral Technique

Landmark: zygomatic arch and tragus.

Injection site: 1 cm below the midpoint of the zygomatic arch or 1 cm anterior to the tragus.

Direction: perpendicular to the skin.

Technique: needle is advanced to a depth of 3 cm towards the base of the infratemporal fossa.

Solution: 3 mL 0.5% bupivacaine with 1 mL Depo-Medrol

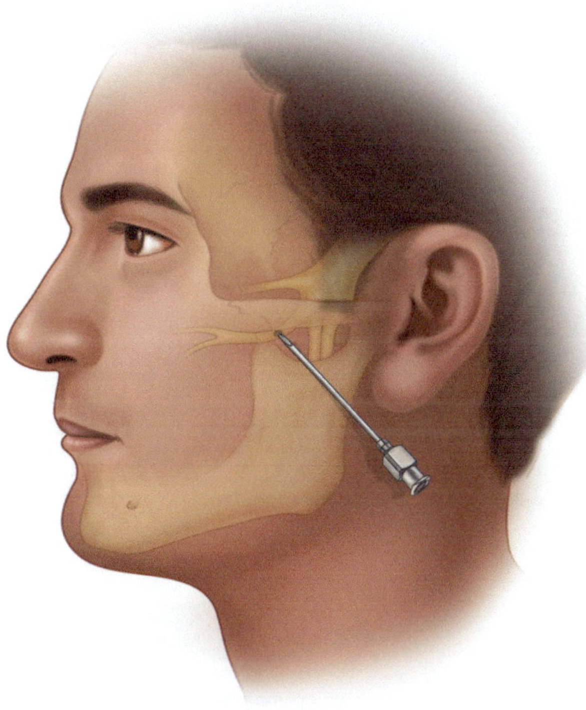

Fig. 14.2 Extraoral technique

Closed-Mouth Technique (Vazirani-Akinosi)

Landmark: gingivo-buccal reflection of mucosa of the upper jaw.

Injection site: behind the last molar and 1 cm above the gingivo-buccal reflection.

Direction: parallel to the occlusal surface.

Technique: needle is advanced for 2 cm against the ramus of the mandible with bevel pointing medially.

Solution: 2 mL of 0.5 % bupivacaine with 1 mL Depo-Medrol

Good oral hygiene plays more than an aesthetic role. It avoids infection which could lead to inflammation and fibrosis. In addition it ensures that the patient has a good appetite and therefore good nutrition. We encourage mouth gargles with any antiseptic solution at least ten times a day. In addition the nursing staff physically cleans oral cavity of the patient with gauze soaked in antiseptic. Addition of H_2O_2 helps to remove slough and food debris if any.

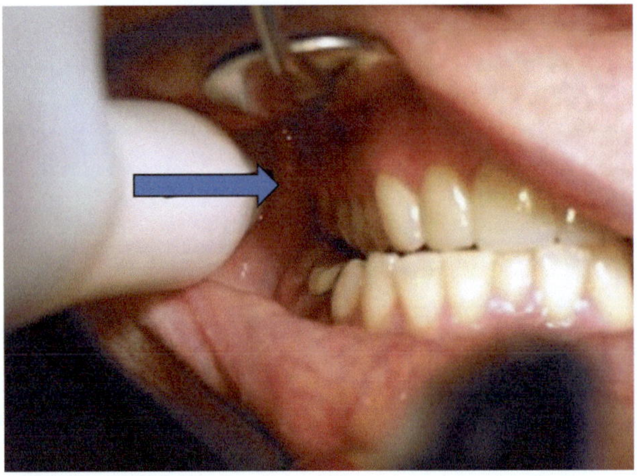

Fig. 14.3 Closed mouth technique

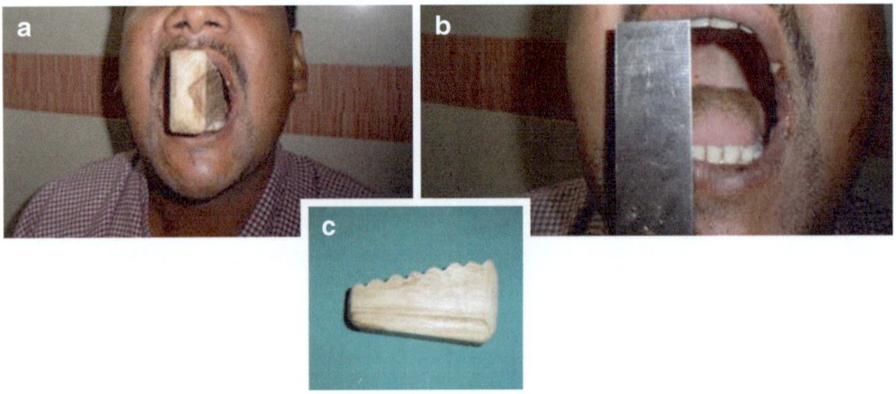

Fig. 14.4 (**a–c**) Use of mouth opening block for mouth opening exercises

Mouth-opening exercises. The role of mouth-opening exercises cannot be overemphasized. They are started right from first postoperative day. There are commercial devices available, like the mouth-opening screw. But they are expensive. We use indigenously designed wooden blocks with slots at 5 mm distance. Using them the patient can themselves quantify the results and get motivated. In the initial stages, patient can even use their own hands with fingers of each hand on upper and lower incisors, pushing the lower incisors down. This has to be performed at least ten times in a day under the close supervision of nursing staff or patient's attendant.

In addition exercises are advised to increase the activity of cheeks by blowing balloons.

Evolution of Surgery of Trismus of OSMF

15

Madan Kapre and Sudhanshu Kothe

Key Points

- Abstinence from habit of chewing tobacco is the most overriding factor in outcomes.
- During our experience of more than three decades, treatment has progressed from medical management only to advanced surgical release and complex flap reconstructions.
- Our "here-to-stay" procedures include double cuts, laser release, extensive release and excision, coronoidectomy, mandibular mucoperiosteal flap, palatal flap, and the platysma flap.

We have been working over last three decades on various surgical options and critically auditing our own work. We have begun with medical management of all sorts including topical injections of numerous types. Results were similar to placebo procedures and are disappointing.

Abstinence from habit of chewing tobacco or betel nut seems to be the most overriding factor, and hence the first lesson was learnt—no surgical intervention for at least 3 months of abstinence from the habit. This also allows to draw the baseline for gradation of trismus. Improvement that occurs with such simple basic measures is a reality and could give false impression about the efficacy of the procedure.

M. Kapre, F.R.C.S., D.L.O. (✉)
Neeti Clinics, Neeti Gaurav Complex, Central Bazar Road, Ramdaspeth, Nagpur, Maharashtra, India
e-mail: madankapre@gmail.com

S. Kothe, M.S., M.Ch., D.N.B.
Department of Plastic and Reconstructive Surgery, Jai Clinics and Neeti Clinics, Nagpur, Maharashtra, India
e-mail: sudhanshu.kothe@gmail.com

M. Kapre, S. Kothe (eds.), *Surgery of Trismus in Oral Submucous Fibrosis*,
https://doi.org/10.1007/978-981-10-4892-0_15

Although we have critically analyzed the various surgical procedures in appropriate sections of this atlas, we present some pearls and suggest guidelines to choose the appropriate procedure for a given case.

Topical application and local injections of proteolytic enzymes or steroids can be best summed up as our own time of assessing our grounds. Our walking years were when we were trying local quick-heal techniques like skin grafts and fat flaps. Now we mention this only to be condemned. Acquiring CO_2 laser added the technique of two parallel cuts but with limited applicability.

CO_2 laser no doubt gives you that little extra precision and relatively less blood to fuzz your incisions. We find CO_2 laser an extremely valuable asset in getting less pain, less bleeding, and relatively less scarring.

The cornerstone to success is good, and adequate mandibular mucoperiosteal flap in the late twentieth century and later, redesigning it early this century, has revolutionized our results. We feel this is undoubtedly the quick heal of our choice. Myocutaneous or myofascial platysma flap opened up a new vista and allowed us to carry out more extensive trismus release procedures. These methods of reconstruction are almost "here-to-stay-forever" procedure for us.

Pearls in surgical procedure:

- Thorough nutritional and medical assessment helps.
- Patient motivation must be validated by a good psychiatric profiling of the patient.
- Reassuring and sympathetic family support is extremely desirable.
- Postoperative pain management will help oral hygiene and physiotherapy.
- Choice of drugs and appropriate nerve blocks will decide your results beyond your surgical procedures.
- We recommend following procedures for the grades of trismus:
- Grade I: two parallel laser-assisted cuts
- Grade II–III: release of trismus with coronoidectomy with either mandibular mucoperiosteal flap or palatal flap
- Grade IV and more: all of the above and reconstruct with platysma myocutaneous flap
- **Conclusion**: If we were to conclude this atlas with our own philosophy, we will ask you to submit to your own passionate commitment as it will override all the obstacles. Scarcity of literature compounded by dogmas of senior colleagues has often put off younger aspirant from undertaking these surgeries. Do explore all the possible surgical techniques but settle down quickly in your own comfort zone and develop your own strategies. Above all talk to people with your audited results as the last words in surgical management of trismus of OSMF are far from said.